Weight Watchers™

THE COMPLETE
DIET BOOK

S I M O N & S C H U S T E R

LONDON·SYDNEY·NEW YORK·TOKYO·SINGAPORE·TORONTO

First published in Great Britain by Simon & Schuster Ltd, 1994
A Paramount Communications Company

Simon & Schuster Ltd
West Garden Place
Kendal Street
London W2 2AQ

Created and produced by
SP Creative Design
147 Kings Road
Bury St Edmunds
Suffolk IP33 3DJ

Written by Heather Thomas
Art Director: Al Rockall
Designer: Rolando Ugolini
Production: Fiona Cannel Finch, Wendy Martin
Photography: Steve Lee, Steve Shipman

Weight Watchers Products Manager: Annette Stribling
Weight Watchers Publications Executive: Delia Bintley

A CIP catalogue record for this book is available from the British Library

ISBN 0-671-71346-9

Typeset in
Stone Serif by Halcyon Type & Design, Ipswich

Printed and bound in Italy by
A. Mondadori, Verona

Acknowledgements

Weight Watchers (UK) Ltd would like to thank the following individuals for their help
in compiling this book:
Medical Advisers: Dr Arnold Bender, Dr Peter Kopelman
Exercise Consultants: Derrick Evans, Kathy Fulcher
Celia Whiston, Judy Clark, Lynn Little, Lynne Macmillan and Margaret Turner
All Members and their Leaders, who are featured in this book

Contents

Ten years ago I made one of the biggest decisions of my life: I gave up dieting. After twenty years of crash diets I had had enough. You are probably thinking that I just gave in to my increasing weight problem, but that's not true. Yes, I did forget about dieting; I joined Weight Watchers, because as this book will teach you, Weight Watchers is not a diet but a healthy eating plan for the rest of your life.

I'm sure that my story will be all too familiar to a lot of you reading this. As a child I was skinny, always active, quite a tomboy in fact. Then I hit my mid teens – I discovered boys, food and a burgeoning weight problem, all in quick succession. This was the start of my 'battle of the bulge', and for the next twenty years I tried every diet ever published, and a few more besides. None of them ever really worked. I became expert at the 'special occasion diet'. I would deprive myself for weeks before a holiday or big night out and normally manage to squeeze into my bikini or dress. Then, as a reward for my success, I would eat everything I had been denying myself and put on all the weight I had lost and usually a bit more too!

In 1981, just before the birth of Emily, my eldest daughter, I gave up work. Without the structure of the office routine my eating habits went completely haywire. I was never really hungry in the morning; in fact, usually I didn't eat anything at all until 3.00pm, but then I would find myself nibbling constantly until I went to bed. Less than a year after Emily was born I was pregnant again, this time with twins. Brilliant, I thought, now I can eat for

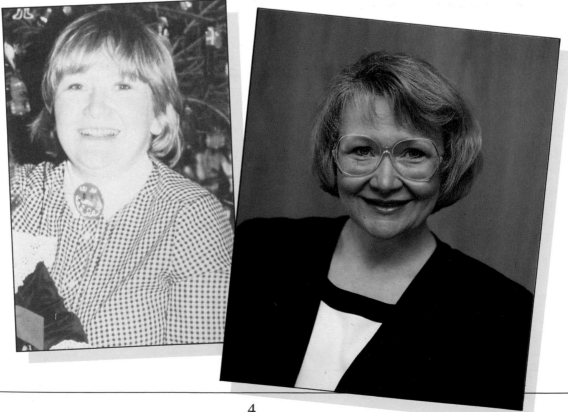

three! During that pregnancy I gained 5½ stone and after the twins were born 3½ stone was still there!

I managed to lose the first 1½ stone by myself but it was a real struggle. I had to admit it, I just wasn't going to make it alone.

From the minute I walked into that first Meeting it just seemed so easy; within 16 weeks I had lost 2 stone and reached my Goal Weight. I think that it was the support I received from other Members that helped me the most: I discovered that I wasn't the only person in the world who could eat a whole cheesecake while it was still frozen, or demolish an entire packet of biscuits just to disguise the fact that I had eaten one or two – what a relief! I love food and I always will but Weight Watchers has taught me how to control it, instead of it controlling me.

When I reached my Goal Weight I decided that I would like to help other people the way Weight Watchers had helped me. All of our Leaders and Managers are successful slimmers with Weight Watchers and so I applied to become a Leader, never dreaming that ten years later I would be Vice President of the company. I can truthfully say that when I lost my weight I gained a whole new life.

Weight Watchers was started for people like you and me by people just like us. Back in 1963 Jean Nidetch, who founded the company in America, was an overweight housewife who started using her friends as a support system to help her lose weight. Jean's 'cookie confessions' gradually grew into weekly meetings and now they cover the whole world, from Hong Kong to Finland. Although our Programme has changed over the years to fit in with all the latest reports and government findings, the basic principles will always be the same as they were 30 years ago – normal, healthy eating with all the support and encouragement that friends can give you.

I hope that this book will offer you exactly that. Weight Watchers has helped over 25 million people lose weight; they did it and I did it . . . you can too!

Linda Huett

LINDA HUETT
VICE PRESIDENT

"I love food and always will but Weight Watchers taught me how to control my weight instead of it controlling me"

The best diet of all is a diet for life, a sensible, balanced approach to eating which will help you lose excess pounds and maintain a healthy weight. This is exactly what the Weight Watchers Programme is, not just a diet but a whole new way of life. Have you tried dieting in the past, only to regain any weight lost as soon as you returned to your old eating habits? This sort of yo-yo dieting is not only bad for your health but can be very demoralizing.

For over thirty years, Weight Watchers has helped millions of people to lose weight and stay slim. Our Programme will teach you how to change your eating habits for good, and this new healthy regime, along with stepping up your level of exercise, will soon have that excess weight literally melting away.

For this book we have devised a special 14-day plan of diet and exercise, which, along with handy slimming hints and advice will show you just how easy losing weight and, even more importantly, keeping it off, can be.

We are the experts in weight loss, and we have developed a unique system which is extremely flexible and enables you to *enjoy* your food and create satisfying delicious meals for you and your family. Now you too will find that dieting really can be fun.

Why are you overweight?

Statistics show that 45 per cent of men and 36 per cent of women in the United Kingdom today are overweight, so you are not alone.

Weight gain is caused by eating more than your body needs.

Although you can control the amount of food you eat, there is one thing that is beyond your control – your genetic make-up. If your parents or grandparents were overweight, there may be a greater chance that you have a tendency to put on weight. However, environmental influences and the eating and exercise patterns you've learned throughout your life, beginning in childhood, can have greater effects on your adult body weight. However, you don't have to accept this as your fate.

TRUDY GREENWOOD

Trudy Greenwood lost an incredible 5 stone and won the Weight Watchers 1992 Success of the Year Competition. Trudy had struggled with her weight for years since she became pregnant with James, her nine-year-old son. "I ate whenever I felt like it, and put on 4 stone. I had this image of all the weight miraculously disappearing after the birth. It came as a bit of a shock when it was still there!"

Trudy continued to put on weight with her other two children, Hollie and Sam, and overeating became a way of life. However, she was becoming increasingly concerned about her weight and tried several 'miracle' diets but without success.

"It took nine years of being overweight to realise that Weight Watchers held the key to my slimmer body. I knew I had to find out about healthy, nutritious food. It was a very big step going to that first Weight Watchers Meeting, but I realised for the first time that I was not alone. The support I received from my Leader and other Members in my group really did contribute to my success."

Trudy found it difficult to accept the

You can do something positive about it, and this book will help to motivate you and set you on the path to long-term permanent weight loss. It is also a well-known fact that the types of food you enjoyed as a child will influence the types of food that you choose to eat as an adult. By changing your eating habits, you will achieve success.

Exercise your options

In addition to being careful about what you eat, you must try to introduce more exercise into your daily routine. With this in mind, we have devised a complete home work-out for you which focuses on those problem areas such as the hips, thighs, bottom and stomach. If you are unused to exercise and lead a very sedentary life, you can make a start just by climbing the stairs instead of using the lift or escalator; or by walking or cycling to the shops instead of taking the car or a bus. Remember any calories you consume which are not burned up

STATISTICS: TRUDY	
AGE:	31
HEIGHT:	5 feet 8 inches
WAS:	15 stone 10 pounds
NOW:	10 stone 11 pounds
LOST:	4 stone 13 pounds

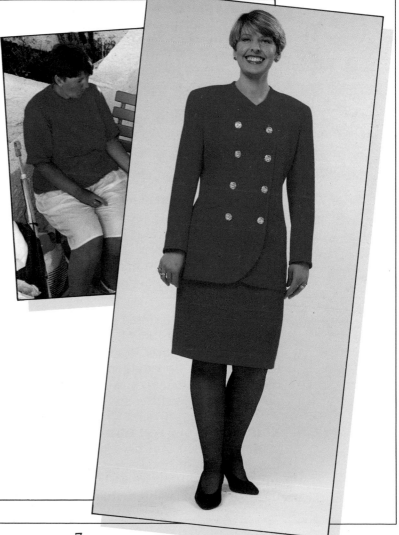

fact that on the Weight Watchers Programme she could have so much to eat. "I felt I needed to deprive myself in order to get slim and stay that way. I now recognise that if I keep on eating a sensible diet, I have a plan for success for the rest of my life."

Losing weight has transformed Trudy's whole life. Now she has a wonderful job caring for disabled people. She goes to aerobic classes three times a week, and joins in all the family outings. Her whole family has benefited too, and they have all adopted more healthy eating habits. Trudy has resolved to stay slim and keep the weight off for good. "I'm so happy with myself, it's been a long time since I felt like that. I'm a happier person so it's better for the family. I'm easier to live with, and I join in all the children's activities now. I'm having too good a time to ever put back the weight I lost!"

BOB GRIFFIN

It took Bob Griffin only a few months to lose an amazing 5 stone and to become Weight Watchers 1992 Male Success of the Year. His only regret was that it took him so long to admit the awful truth to himself – that he was overweight! "I never realised just how gross I'd got, because people used to say, 'You're just a big lad' and 'You carry it well,' so it never really bothered me."

During the eight years of their marriage before Bob joined Weight Watchers, his wife Glenda had watched his weight creep up to a hefty 19 stone, and she had witnessed him trying the various diets and slimming aids that always failed miserably.

Bob realises now that eating all the wrong kinds of foods led to his weight gain at school, but the pounds were creeping up slowly and he refused to notice that he was getting bigger. By the time his second child was born, he was finding it difficult to perform even the simplest of tasks, like bending down to wash his feet in the shower!

However, the strain of being overweight started to get to Bob. "As I was getting bigger, I didn't actually weigh myself, I just bought bigger clothes. It got to the point though where clothes weren't available off-the-peg and that was embarrassing – it drove it home to me that I was an outsize person. Even though you try to hide how you feel, inside you know that you should do something about it."

STATISTICS: BOB	
AGE:	37
HEIGHT:	6 feet 1½ inches
WAS:	19 stone 3 pounds
NOW:	14 stone 1½ pounds
LOST:	5 stone 1½ pounds

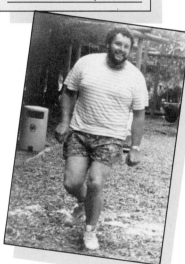

during the day are stored as fat in your body. Don't worry about having to exercise if you've never done it before. Initially it can be very gentle and you can gradually increase the amount you do as you become fitter and slimmer.

You need never feel hungry!

With most diets you have to count all the calories in the food you eat each day, and one of the problems with this is that there is no guarantee that you are getting a nutritionally balanced diet. The Weight Watchers Programme is different: there is no calorie counting nor do you have to eat a strictly controlled diet with an inflexible daily food plan. On the 14-day Programme in this book (see page 118) we give you a menu to follow every day.

It is important that when you follow the Programme you eat three satisfying meals a day. This means you need never feel hungry or 'go without'. In fact,

The time had come to act. Thankfully, Glenda had seen an advertisement for Weight Watchers in a newspaper, and so Bob went along to a Meeting, and he's never looked back! "It came as a huge shock when I was standing on the scales and I was told how much I weighed. Initially I thought, 'I've got to lose over 5 stone', and it seemed like an impossible task. But the encouragement was there, and the first week I came back I'd lost 12 pounds. Then it really got a grip on me, and I really wanted to lose weight. I knew it could be done – the second week I lost 8 pounds."

In the early days Bob was teased by his male friends about joining Weight Watchers, but he knew that he needed help in losing weight; he couldn't do it on his own. "I needed help, and I needed guidance, which I got from Weight Watchers."

Bob changed his eating habits for good and even started jogging, and now he feels fitter and healthier than he has for a long time. His workmates stopped teasing him when they saw the results of his endeavours. Bob's whole family has benefited from his success, and he is determined to stay a fit and active father and husband.

some people comment that they have never eaten so much!

Does being overweight really matter?

How many times have you heard it said that it is better to be overweight and happy than thin and miserable? Both research and Weight Watchers Members tell us that most overweight people would prefer to be slim. Being significantly overweight can influence your health adversely. It can increase the risk of developing the following:

- Cardiovascular disease
- Diabetes
- High blood pressure
- Gall bladder disease
- Arthritis
- Complications during surgery

Being significantly overweight is bad for your health, physically and mentally.

If you are self-conscious about your size it is easy to become depressed. Overhearing remarks in the street, or being teased about your size can really lower your self-esteem. You're less likely to feel like going out and socializing, and a general lack of self-confidence will affect your work. If you recognise these feelings, don't despair. You can do something positive to lose weight, and as you're losing it, just remember what you will be gaining!

- You will feel better about yourself
- You will feel healthier
- You will feel more attractive
- You will increase your self-esteem
- You will eat a healthier diet
- You can wear more fashionable clothes

Who says that being overweight does not really matter? Most people realise that they will feel better when they are fit, healthy and slim rather than when they are carrying around excess pounds.

Change your life now!

Here at Weight Watchers, we know that most of our Members enjoy food, love eating and like cooking. Diets that are

I can do it!

biased heavily towards making sacrifices and going without won't work in the long term because people don't want to deny themselves the foods they enjoy so much. They do want to enjoy their favourite foods in moderation and to eat a varied diet – in other words, to learn to eat normally. Once you start to explore your relationship with food, you will be able to identify both the 'danger' situations that you get into and those problem foods that prove irresistible.

Recognising these things is one of the first steps to taking control of your weight, and your life. Remember:

- You **can** still eat well
- You **can** still eat out
- You **can** plan your own meals
- You **can** decide what you eat – and how much
- You **can** do it – and you **will** be successful

MANDY HILL

Mandy Hill had been overweight since childhood, and had tried many diets unsuccessfully, but now she is slim for the first time in her life, thanks to Weight Watchers. Mandy's trouble was that she loved food too much to stop eating; she thought that dieting meant giving up all the food she enjoyed and feeling hungry. "But of course I learned that you don't have to. In fact, much to my surprise, I ate really well on the Weight Watchers Programme. There's lot of choices of breakfasts, light meals and main meals."

Mandy lost 4 stone in total on the Programme. "You wouldn't believe the difference in me now. For a start, I like myself and believe in myself. I've got a new job, I'm wearing lovely fashionable clothes which I never could have worn before, and I really feel healthy for the first time."

She understands how difficult it is to do something about being overweight because she has felt like that most of her life. "What I'd like to say to others who need to lose weight is that once you get started it's not that difficult because you can still really enjoy your food." Mandy did it . . . and so can you!

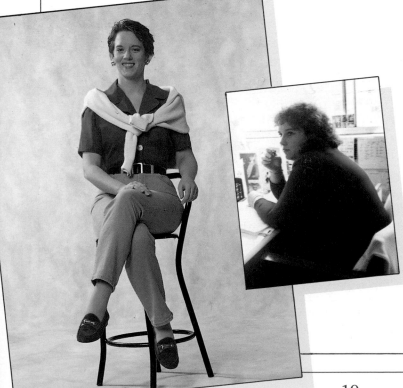

STATISTICS: MANDY	
AGE: 26	
HEIGHT: 5 feet 6 inches	
WAS: 14 stone ¾ pound	
NOW: 10 stone	
LOST: 4 stone ¾ pound	

10

LESLEY BAINES

Before glamorous Lesley Baines joined Weight Watchers, she was over 15 stone, suffered from high blood pressure and bad joints, and was fed up with her appearance as well as her health. One year later, she was a trim 9 stone 8 pounds.

Looking back to that time, Lesley recalls: "My joints were getting so bad I had to strap up my ankles so I could walk. Just a short walk to the bus stop left me puffing and panting, and I found it difficult to bend down."

It is no wonder that Lesley felt depressed, and when her husband Paul decided to take her to a charity ball to cheer her up, Lesley treated herself to a new ballgown. However, the one she chose, a size 26 in a shiny ruched material, only drew attention to her weight problem. When she saw a photo of herself afterwards, she was horrified and took the decision that changed her life: she decided to join Weight Watchers.

Her first two weeks were the worst because she used to eat several chocolate bars a day, and she felt very low when she reduced her sugar intake.

She started exercising when she reached 14 stone and became more mobile. She had a fitness assessment at a local gym and embarked on a gentle exercise programme. "I enjoyed it so much I ended up going seven days a week. I loved it and got absolutely hooked. I started off with a low-impact version because my joints wouldn't stand up to any pounding."

Lesley loved exercising so much that now she is slim and 5 stone 7 pounds lighter, she still continues to work out and is now a trained fitness instructor herself. "I love the feeling that it gives me. Exercise is something I could never

STATISTICS: LESLEY	
AGE:	35
HEIGHT:	5 feet 5 inches
WAS:	15 stone 1 pound
NOW:	9 stone 8 pounds
LOST:	5 stone 7 pounds

do before, and now I'm making up for all those lost years. It gives me a wonderful feeling of freedom. If you're fit, you enjoy life more."

Lesley lost weight so successfully that she was persuaded to enter the 1989/90 Weight Watchers Member of the Year competition, and she won! "When I lost the weight, I discovered that there was a slim body inside the old fat me. My life has changed completely. I exercise most days. I eat healthily and well: a lot of food, so I don't starve myself. I'm in control of my eating and my body now, and I feel better about myself than I did at sixteen!. My motto is everything in moderation, and then I'm in control of my whole life."

The factors to take into account when choosing your target weight are your sex, age, height, build and body shape. The charts opposite will give you your particular healthy weight range, and ideally you should select a weight from within this band. You should select a target weight which you feel is attainable. You can always adjust it when you see just how easy it is to lose those excess pounds. Remember, though, that you must not go below the minimum weight in your range. It is unhealthy to be too thin.

The best way to lose weight – and to keep it off long term – is to lose it slowly and steadily. Some people are so impatient to lose weight and see rapid results that they embark on dangerous crash diets. They may lose a lot of weight quickly, but the pounds will soon pile back on, and the likelihood is that they will end up in a never-ending cycle of dieting and weight gain.

Keeping a personal weight loss chart

It is a good idea to keep a personal weight loss chart to record your weight loss and how successful you are. Every week you can jot your new weight down on the chart, together with your measurements, once a fortnight, e.g. your hips, thighs, knees, chest, upper arms and waist. It will be very motivating to see the inches literally disappear and to look back to your original weight and measurements and congratulate yourself on the progress you have made.
● Around the thickest part of your upper arms
● Loosely around your waist
● Around the fullest part of your chest or bust
● Around the fullest part of your hips and bottom
● Around the fullest part of your thighs
● Loosely around your knees

How many people do you know who always seem to be on a diet? The chances are that they are caught in the vicious cycle of dieting and overeating which never leads to permanent weight loss. However, patience is the name of the game and after an initial weight loss that will delight you in the first couple of weeks or so, you will find that your weekly loss will even out to a steady 1 to 2 pounds. Don't be disappointed when this happens; medical experts tell us that losing 1 to 2 pounds a week is the safest and most successful way to diet.

Everybody loses weight at a different rate, and your personal weight loss is dependent on several factors: how much food you were eating before you started your diet; how closely you follow the Programme; how effectively you measure and weigh the food you eat; how much exercise you take; and, of course, how determined you are to succeed.

Weight lost steadily will bring dividends in the future, helping you to maintain your new figure and bringing long-term success. It is easy to get frustrated if you have a lot to lose and the pounds are not shifting quickly enough, or you cannot *see* the results in your shape and figure even when the scales are reading less. However, don't despair! This is where Weight Watchers Meetings could really help you. If you go along to a Meeting, you will meet other people who are in a similar situation to you and facing all the same problems. By making the most of their moral support, you can help each other to lose weight.

Check your weight loss

You should only weigh yourself once a

HEALTHY WEIGHT RANGE

IN STONES AND POUNDS FOR MEN AND WOMEN

HEIGHT Without shoes in ft. in	MIN JOINING WEIGHT in st. lb.	WOMEN 16 - 25 Years Healthy Range	WOMEN 26 - 45 Years Healthy Range	WOMEN 45 Years + Healthy Range	MEN 16 Years and over Healthy Range	Max allowed	HEIGHT Without shoes in metres
4' 6"	6.11	6.1 - 6.9	6.1 - 6.12	6.1 - 7.2	6.1 - 7.6	8.1	1.37m
4' 7"	6.12	6.2 - 6.12	6.2 - 7.1	6.2 - 7.6	6.2 - 7.10	8.5	1.40m
4' 8"	7.0	6.4 - 7.2	6.4 - 7.5	6.4 - 7.10	6.4 - 8.0	8.9	1.42m
4' 9"	7.4	6.8 - 7.5	6.8 - 7.9	6.8 - 8.0	6.8 - 8.4	8.13	1.45m
4' 10"	7.7	6.11 - 7.9	6.11 - 7.13	6.11 - 8.3	6.11 - 8.8	9.4	1.47m
4' 11"	7.10	7.0 - 7.12	7.0 - 8.3	7.0 - 8.7	7.0 - 8.12	9.9	1.50m
5' 0"	8.0	7.4 - 8.2	7.4 - 8.7	7.4 - 8.11	7.4 - 9.2	10.0	1.52m
5' 1"	8.3	7.7 - 8.5	7.7 - 8.10	7.7 - 9.1	7.7 - 9.7	10.5	1.55m
5' 2"	8.6	7.10 - 8.9	7.10 - 9.0	7.7 - 9.1	7.7 - 9.7	10.8	1.57m
5' 3"	8.9	7.13 - 8.13	7.13 - 9.4	7.10 - 9.6	7.10 - 9.11	10.13	1.60m
5' 4"	8.12	8.2 - 9.3	8.2 - 9.8	7.13 - 9.10	7.13 - 10.2	11.4	1.63m
5' 5"	9.2	8.6 - 9.7	8.6 - 9.13	8.2 - 10.0	8.2 - 10.6	11.9	1.65m
5' 6"	9.6	8.10 - 9.11	8.10 - 10.3	8.6 - 10.5	8.6 - 10.10	12.0	1.68m
5' 7"	9.10	9.0 - 10.1	9.0 - 10.7	8.10 - 10.10	8.10 - 11.1	12.5	1.70m
5' 8"	10.0	9.4 - 10.5	9.4 - 10.12	9.0 - 11.1	9.0 - 11.6	12.10	1.73m
5' 9"	10.4	9.8 - 10.9	9.8 - 11.2	9.4 - 11.6	9.4 - 11.11	13.1	1.75m
5' 10"	10.8	9.12 - 11.0	9.12 - 11.7	9.8 - 11.10	9.8 - 12.2	13.7	1.78m
5' 11"	10.12	10.2 - 11.4	10.2 - 11.12	9.12 - 12.0	9.12 - 12.6	13.13	1.80m
6' 0"	11.2	10.6 - 11.9	10.6 - 12.3	10.2 - 12.5	10.2 - 12.12	14.5	1.83m
6' 1"	11.6	10.10 - 12.0	10.10 - 12.8	10.6 - 12.9	10.6 - 13.2	14.11	1.85m
6' 2"	11.10	11.0 - 12.4	11.0 - 12.12	10.10 - 13.0	10.10 - 13.7	15.3	1.88m
				11.0 - 13.5	11.0 - 13.13		

IN KILOGRAMMES FOR MEN AND WOMEN

HEIGHT Without shoes in metres	MIN JOINING WEIGHT in kg	WOMEN 16 - 25 Years Healthy Range	WOMEN 26 - 45 Years Healthy Range	WOMEN 45 Years + Healthy Range	MEN 16 Years and over Healthy Range	Max allowed	HEIGHT Without shoes in ft. in.
1.37m	43.1	38.6 - 42.2	38.6 - 43.6	38.6 - 45.4	38.6 - 47.2	51.3	4' 6"
1.40m	43.5	39.0 - 43.6	39.0 - 44.9	39.0 - 47.2	39.0 - 49.0	53.1	4' 7"
1.42m	44.5	39.9 - 45.4	39.9 - 46.7	39.9 - 49.0	39.9 - 50.8	54.9	4' 8"
1.45m	46.2	41.7 - 46.7	41.7 - 48.5	41.7 - 50.8	41.7 - 52.6	56.7	4' 9"
1.47m	47.6	43.1 - 48.5	43.1 - 50.4	43.1 - 52.2	43.1 - 54.4	59.0	4' 10"
1.50m	49.0	44.5 - 49.9	44.5 - 52.2	44.5 - 54.0	44.5 - 56.3	61.2	4' 11"
1.52m	50.8	46.3 - 51.7	46.3 - 54.0	46.3 - 55.8	46.3 - 58.0	63.5	5' 0"
1.55m	52.1	47.6 - 53.1	47.6 - 55.3	47.6 - 57.6	47.6 - 60.3	65.8	5' 1"
1.57m	53.5	49.0 - 54.9	49.0 - 57.2	49.0 - 59.9	49.0 - 62.1	67.1	5' 2"
1.60m	54.9	50.4 - 56.7	50.4 - 59.0	50.4 - 61.7	50.4 - 64.4	69.4	5' 3"
1.63m	56.2	51.7 - 58.5	51.7 - 60.8	51.7 - 63.5	51.7 - 66.2	71.7	5' 4"
1.65m	58.0	53.5 - 60.3	53.5 - 63.1	53.5 - 65.8	53.5 - 68.0	73.9	5' 5"
1.68m	59.8	55.3 - 62.1	55.3 - 64.9	55.3 - 68.0	55.3 - 70.3	76.2	5' 6"
1.70m	61.7	57.2 - 64.0	57.2 - 66.7	57.2 - 70.3	57.2 - 72.6	78.5	5' 7"
1.73m	63.5	59.0 - 65.8	59.0 - 69.0	59.0 - 72.6	59.0 - 74.8	80.7	5' 8"
1.75m	65.3	60.8 - 67.6	60.8 - 70.8	60.8 - 74.4	60.8 - 77.1	83.0	5' 9"
1.78m	67.1	62.6 - 69.9	62.6 - 73.0	62.6 - 76.2	62.6 - 78.9	85.7	5' 10"
1.80m	68.9	64.4 - 71.7	64.4 - 75.3	64.4 - 78.5	64.4 - 81.7	88.5	5' 11"
1.83m	70.7	66.2 - 73.9	66.2 - 77.6	66.2 - 80.3	66.2 - 83.5	91.2	6' 0"
1.85m	72.5	68.0 - 76.2	68.0 - 79.8	66.2 - 80.3	66.2 - 83.5	93.9	6' 1"
1.88m	74.4	69.9 - 78.0	69.9 - 81.7	68.0 - 82.6	68.0 - 85.7	96.6	6' 2"
				69.9 - 84.8	69.9 - 88.5		

week, using accurate scales. Your weight can fluctuate from day to day, as well as throughout the day, so you should try to weigh yourself under the same conditions. Note also that for women, weight can vary at different times of the menstrual cycle.

Weighing yourself

● Weigh yourself at the same time of day, e.g. first thing in the morning before you eat breakfast

● Weigh yourself on the same set of scales in the same place

● Wear similar clothes when you weigh yourself

● Weigh just once a week and resist the temptation to keep hopping on the scales – you may get disappointed if you can't see any difference, or your weight loss is proceeding too slowly; or you may be tempted to 'reward' yourself if you're doing well, which can be equally damaging

What body shape am I?

Are you an apple or a pear? That may sound like a silly question but this is how experts now distinguish between different body shapes. Women tend to be pear shaped with most of their fat distributed around their hips, whereas most overweight men fall into the apple-shaped category with the bulk of their fat around their waist, but each sex can be either shape. Traditionally, body types are categorized as:

1 Ectomorphs: You have narrow shoulders and hips.

2 Mesomorphs: You have broad shoulders and narrow hips.

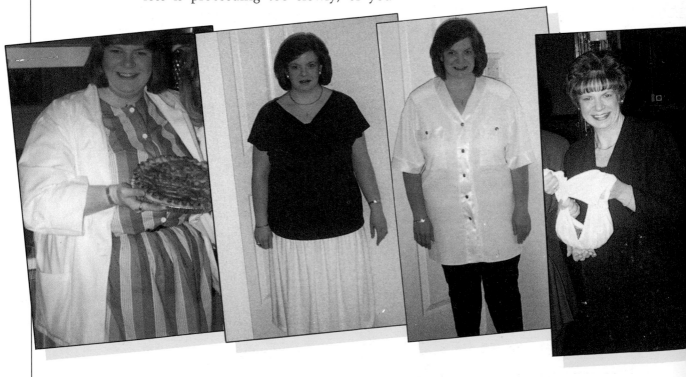

JEAN WALKER

Jean Walker recorded her incredible weight loss of 7 stone 6 pounds by taking photographs of herself every month. "I took the photos so I could see how much weight I was losing. They are a reminder to me of what I used to be like, and will help motivate me to stay slim in the future."

Jean had always been overweight. Her father was a baker and she was brought up on pies and pastries. She decided to join Weight Watchers after a friend asked her to be her bridesmaid. "I wasn't happy with myself, and deep down inside I wanted to be slim."

Jean was determined to succeed, and she changed her eating habits completely. "The first thing I did was to get rid of the deep-fat fryer; I grilled everything instead. I found that I ate much more interesting food, and if I felt hungry, I filled up on vegetables and diet coke, or I chewed some sugar-free gum."

Jean lost weight steadily – about 1½ to 2 pounds per week. She started exercising to help speed up her weight loss, and used her exercise bike every night. She even took up badminton.

She is confident that she can stay at her goal. "I'm very happy about the way I am now. In the past, I used to feel left out when there were outings and social events, but now I can join in, and I feel a lot better in myself. I'm determined to stay slim – the photos will see to that!"

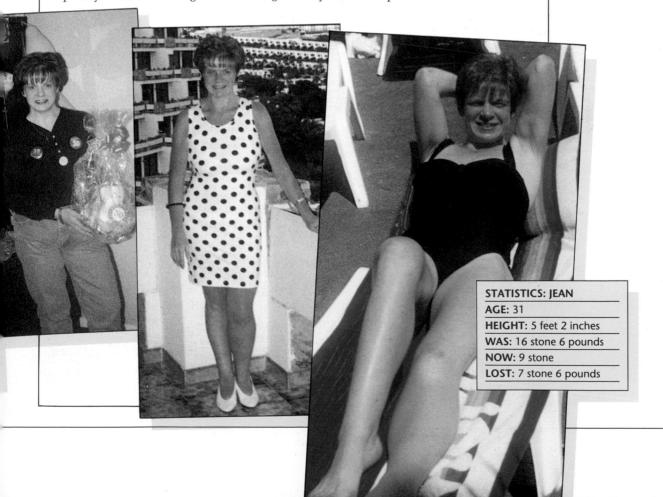

STATISTICS: JEAN	
AGE: 31	
HEIGHT: 5 feet 2 inches	
WAS: 16 stone 6 pounds	
NOW: 9 stone	
LOST: 7 stone 6 pounds	

Keep a photo weight loss record

When you finally make the decision to follow our Programme and change to new healthier eating habits, it is a good idea to get someone to take a full-length photo of you, and then continue taking photographs at monthly intervals and watch the transformation in your shape as the weight rolls off and you slim down. You will be amazed at the difference that just a few pounds can make.

If you hit a bad patch when your weight loss seems to have slowed down and you may be getting impatient and frustrated, it will motivate you to continue the good work if you can look back at the photos of how you used to be and see what you have achieved already. You can do it, no matter how far you still have to go.

3 Endomorphs: You have broad shoulders and broad hips.

Which body type are you? Although you can change your figure by slimming and exercise, your basic body shape will always remain the same.

How much weight can I lose safely?

When you embark on our Programme it is important to set yourself a realistic target, as being over-ambitious can easily result in failure and disappointment. Gradual weight loss is the safest way to slim, and if you are generally in good health you can follow our 14-day menu plan and exercise programme outlined in this book without suffering any ill effects. However, it is always a good idea to check with your doctor first.

Crash diets can damage your health, particularly if you try to follow them for more than a limited time. They work on the principle that you reduce your calorie intake to a mere survival level, and burn up many more calories than you take in, thereby losing weight. They may be OK in the short term for a few lucky people with only a few pounds to lose, but they can be very dangerous.

You might think that it does not matter nutritionally how you get your calories, but it does matter a great deal. By following the Weight Watchers Programme you can be confident that you are getting all the goodness you need as you will eat regular meals which include a wide range of foods.

How long will it take?

You may ask yourself: "Will I ever reach my target weight?" The answer is – of course you will! It may take time, and so try not to be impatient. Take it one day at a time, even one hour at a time if necessary. You probably gained the weight over several months or even years, and it will not disappear overnight.

At Weight Watchers, we have no magic cures or gimmicks. If you have a large amount of weight to lose, say, in excess of two stone, it will take time, and the more you have to lose, the longer it may take, but slowly and surely you will be successful. We all want a dieting short-cut, but the only diet that will really work is a diet that you can stick to and enjoy. Gradual weight loss will ensure success and help you to maintain your target weight long term.

NIKKI NUNN

When Nikki Nunn decided to join Weight Watchers, she started to make a photo record of her personal weight loss. In this way, she could see her transformation as the pounds rolled off and she gradually became slimmer.

Nikki had always had problems with her weight since being a teenager, and after two difficult pregnancies when she couldn't exercise, her weight got out of control. She tried various crash diets which seemed to work in the short term, but then the weight would creep back on again.

Nikki lost the first five and a half stone by following the Weight Watchers By Mail Programme at home, losing between one and a half to two pounds per week. "This slow weight loss was better than losing weight rapidly because it was easier to maintain. But then I hit a plateau and didn't achieve any further progress for two to three months. At last I decided to go along to my local Meeting and I was encouraged by my Leader to carry on and eventually achieve my Goal Weight."

Nikki's weakness had always been for sweet food but she enjoyed the Weight Watchers Programme. "You can have a lot more carbohydrates and less protein. It was great for me – I never felt hungry. I knew that here at last was a diet that I could stick to, and maintain."

Now she has reached her goal, Nikki is convinced that this time the weight will stay off, with a combination of healthy food and exercise.

STATISTICS: NIKKI	
AGE:	31
HEIGHT:	5 feet 6 inches
WAS:	17 stone 9 pounds
NOW:	10 stone 1¾ pounds
LOST:	7 stone 7¼ pounds

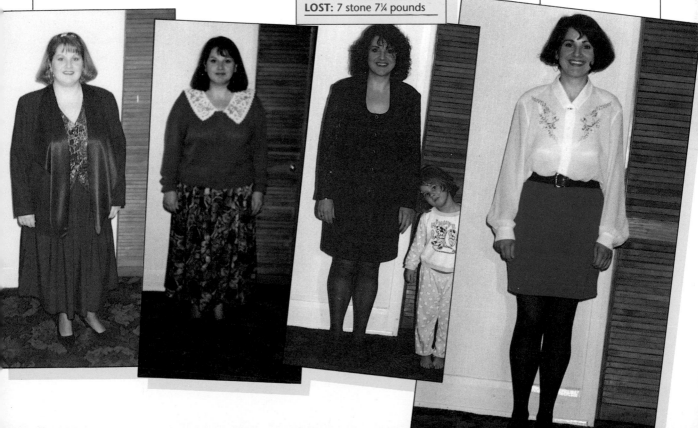

So are you ready? How do you start? You have already taken the most important step by recognising that you have a weight problem and that you want to do something positive about it. Congratulations! Try out our special 14-day diet and exercise programme (see page 118) to get off to a good start. If you want to aim for long-term weight loss, or don't want to go it alone, you can of course join a Weight Watchers Meeting where you will receive support and motivation each week.

Joining Weight Watchers

Every week we hold approximately 3,400 Meetings in the UK alone – all run by Leaders who have lost weight successfully themselves by following the Weight Watchers Programme. They are ideally placed to know how you feel and how best to help you; after all, they have been there themselves. They can understand from their own experience what you are going through, and can offer advice, sympathy and encouragement so that you don't have to go it alone.

Dieting can sometimes seem like a lonely road. It is reassuring to know that if you encounter a problem or a setback there is somebody to whom you can turn, who you can trust and who can understand how you feel. Your fellow Members at the Meeting will provide moral support as well as companionship. You will share experiences, the good and the bad times, the successes and the setbacks. Losing weight can be fun. With the help of your Leader and the other Members you can achieve your goal and be successful. There are thousands of Weight Watchers success stories to inspire you – people of all ages,

nationalities and occupations, all bound together by a shared experience and achievement. You can do it too!

What happens at the Meetings?

Many people who have never attended a Weight Watchers Meeting have some strange notions about what happens, so it is a pleasant surprise for most new Members to realise that they are among friends – all with a common purpose. There is no humiliation and no-one except the Leader knows your weight.

After you have registered on your first visit, you will be weighed and your Leader will discuss a suitable Goal Weight with you. This will be based on several factors: your sex, age and height. At every Meeting, the Leader talks about different aspects of the Programme, nutrition, healthy eating, recipe ideas and exercise. Occasionally, she demonstrates recipes and offers small amounts of food to sample. Members are always invited to ask questions and join in a lively discussion.

Of course, if you feel nervous about speaking out you can just sit back and listen, but you will soon start to feel more confident as you get to know people and lose your inhibitions about discussing your personal experiences.

Your Leader will also answer any questions you may have about the Programme, and advise you on how to deal with difficult eating situations like: what foods to choose when eating out; how to cope at parties; and sticking to your diet when you are away on holiday. She will teach you about the Food Plan, keep a record of your weight loss progress, give you extra support when you need it, and generally motivate and inspire you to succeed.

Where is my local Meeting?

Weight Watchers Meetings are held weekly all over the UK. To find out the details of your nearest Meeting, just phone your local area office as shown on the map at the end of this book, or Weight Watchers Head Office on 0628 777077. You can also look us up in Yellow Pages.

Questions you ask

New Members always have lots of questions they want their Leader to answer – for general information and for reassurance that they are doing the right thing. Here are some of the most commonly asked questions . . . and answers.

"Is Weight Watchers safe?"

Weight Watchers is the world's number one weight loss organisation and since it was founded by Jean Nidetch, in America in 1963, it has helped over 37 million Members throughout the world to lose weight – safely and successfully.

The Programme is updated continually according to the latest nutritional recommendations. There are no fads or gimmicks – just good nutrition. Our Programme is recommended by many doctors and by leading nutritionists because they know that it is nutritionally sound and helps you to lose weight gradually and safely. High in fibre, low in fat, healthy and well-balanced, the Programme reflects current Government recommendations for a healthy way of eating.

What makes the Programme so special is that it is not only designed for you, the dieter, but also for your whole family so that they too can change to a new healthy way of eating and hopefully avoid any weight problems in the future. Real long-term success is built on learning to change your eating habits for good, and the 14-day dieting plan in this book will start you off and build the foundations for future healthy eating.

"Can I afford it?"

Our weight loss Programme is not expensive. There is no need to buy special foods. The foods you will eat are everyday items which will fit comfortably into your weekly budget. You do not need to eat special, exotic meals on the Programme – unless you want to, of course. The Programme is based on poultry, fish, meat, cheese, yogurt and dairy produce, fresh fruit and vegetables and high-fibre cereals – bread, rice and pasta. We have lots of ideas for economy meals, and it is usually possible to substitute a lower-cost food if you wish.

"How much weight can I expect to lose?"

You set your own target weight according to your height, age and sex. You must not expect a rapid weight loss. You will lose weight gradually and steadily. Everybody loses weight at a different pace and your individual weight loss will be determined by such factors as:

● How much food you were eating before you started on the Programme

● How determined you are to lose weight

● Whether you exercise regularly

On average, you should expect to lose 1 to 2 pounds per week, which is a sensible amount to lose. Weight lost slowly is more likely to stay off for good. Crash diets yield a dramatic weight loss in the short term but because most of this loss is fluid, the weight is soon back on again, especially if you do not change your eating habits and recognise why you have a weight problem.

"Will I have to eat differently from the rest of my family?"

No. The Weight Watchers Programme is built on eating ordinary everyday foods that all the family can enjoy. As you learn to prepare and cook nutritious foods in a healthy way, you will change their eating habits, as well as your own, for the better, and especially those of your children. The eating patterns established in childhood are the ones that stay with you throughout your life, and if your children eat nutritious food now, they will grow up into healthy adults.

When the rest of your family discover how delicious the food on the Programme really is, they will be only too anxious to share it with you, although they can of course eat larger portions. You can still enjoy your old favourites like casseroles, grills, roasts, rice and pasta dishes, stir-fries and even desserts, but all made with low-calorie ingredients. You will find lots of interesting recipe ideas in this book to start you off.

"Will I have to change my lifestyle?"

No, but there are two things that you will probably have to change – your eating habits and how often you exercise. We recognise that at different times you may have to adapt the Programme and your eating habits to meet your different needs. This is easy to do because the Programme is very flexible and is based on sensible eating, so you simply adapt the foods you eat at a given time

to meet the requirements of your busy lifestyle.

If you go out to work – no problem! You can still follow our weight loss Programme. Just take a packed lunch of a healthy salad or sandwich with some raw vegetables or fruit or a low-fat yogurt (taken out of your daily allowance). Nothing could be easier.

You will find some delicious ideas for packed lunches later in the book. As long as you eat three meals a day, you will be fine. Each day you will need to have the following:

- A breakfast
- A light meal
- A main meal

The secret of any successful diet is *balance*, and you should spread your daily food intake throughout the day. If you skip meals you will upset this delicate balance and create problem times when you feel hungry and are more likely to succumb to temptation.

"Can vegetarians go on the Weight Watchers Programme?"

Yes. The Weight Watchers Programme is suitable for vegetarians as it is very flexible and allows you to choose the foods you like from specific food groups. As a vegetarian you should take extra care to ensure that you get adequate amounts of protein and other nutrients, but it is perfectly possible to eat a nutritionally sound balanced diet and still lose weight. For more information on vegetarian food and slimming, turn to page 50. There is a special 14-day Vegetarian menu plan starting on page 118.

"Can anyone join a Weight Watchers Meeting?"

You can join Weight Watchers and

AMANDA GIBBS

It was Amanda Gibbs' mother who persuaded her to go to Weight Watchers and lose a staggering 6 stone 11 pounds. Having unsuccessfully tried countless diets, Amanda had virtually given up on the idea of being slim. "My mother had major surgery on her spine and spent six months on her back in terrible pain. The doctor told her that she must lose weight and she wanted to go to Weight Watchers, and for me to go with her. Eventually I gave in and went along."

Taking the first step was hard enough but sticking to the Programme was even harder for Amanda. "I did lose 30 pounds initially and then I was stuck for months and months and I was going to give up, but all of a sudden I got started again and the rest was easy."

Amanda got 'stuck' because she wasn't following the Programme properly, but after a struggle she learned more about food and changed her eating habits. "I would never have believed that I could eat so many vegetables. Before, I could sit and eat three pounds of chocolate; now I don't even feel like eating one bar. Now I know what is in food, I know what to avoid."

Amanda's other big lifestyle change was to go to weekly keep-fit classes, and to work out on her favourite toning tables. She reached Goal Weight in time to fit into her beautiful fitted Chantilly wedding dress. Her waist, which was once 45 inches, reduced to a slim 28½ inches. Amanda even converted Mario, her husband, to eating the Weight Watchers way and now he loves her healthy cooking too.

STATISTICS: AMANDA	
AGE:	28
HEIGHT:	5 feet 8 inches
WAS:	17 stone 7 pounds
NOW:	10 stone 10 pounds
LOST:	6 stone 11 pounds

come to our weekly Meetings if you are a minimum of 10 pounds heavier than the lowest weight in the recommended healthy weight range for your age and height, and want to lose at least 7 pounds. Our Programme is suitable for men, women and teenagers, although young people between 10 and 16 years of age need to get both their parents' and their doctor's written permission to join. Their doctor will help in setting them a target weight. Children under 10 years of age are not eligible.

If you feel overweight, why not go along to your local Meeting and join? You have nothing to lose but weight!

"Will I have to weigh and measure my food?"

Yes. It is very important that you do weigh and measure all the food you eat if you are to be successful in your weight loss quest. You will eat a variety of foods to ensure a safe level of nutrition and must have at least the minimum quantities that we recommend. If you eat too little, you will upset this delicate nutritional balance and might even damage your health. On the other hand, if you eat too much, you will not lose weight.

"Will I have to go without my favourite foods?"

No. No foods are forbidden on the Weight Watchers Programme, and you can still treat yourself to a little of what you fancy, whether it's the occasional bar of chocolate or a glass of wine. We will teach you how to enjoy them in moderation and how to control the way you eat so that you don't feel deprived. In fact, you will be pleasantly surprised at the range of foods you can continue to eat and enjoy while you are losing weight.

"Do I have to exercise?"

You don't *have* to exercise, but if you do it regularly, it will help you to tone and shape your body as you gradually lose the unwanted pounds. As you will see from pages 104 - 117, you don't have to embark on a rigorous exercise regime of high-intensity aerobics, nor need you take up jogging or weight-training nor go for the burn! Regular stretching and toning exercises will help you train without feeling the strain. Start off slowly and make exercise a part of your life and daily routine. Just fifteen to twenty minutes three or four times a week will help you to firm your figure, especially the problem areas like hips, thighs and stomach. You can do the exercises we recommend at home – you don't have to join a gym or exercise class unless you want to do so. You don't need any special equipment and you can perform your exercises at the time of day that suits you best. Remember that when you reach your target weight, regular exercise will help to maintain your weight and keep you slim. Exercise really is good news!

"What if I can't attend Meetings?"

If you can't or don't want to go to Meetings, but feel you still need the support and back-up that Weight Watchers will give you, you could try

EILEEN AND DENISE TAYLOR

Between them, mother and daughter team Eileen and Denise Taylor have lost an amazing 12 stone 11½ pounds since they took the plunge and went along to their local Weight Watchers Meeting.

Eileen joined Weight Watchers to give her daughter Denise some support. She led a very sedentary lifestyle, and over the years her weight had rocketed until she was a size 30. She had virtually no social life, spending all her time indoors, nearly crippled with arthritis.

She says, "I would sit and watch TV all night and day, bingeing on packets of crisps and biscuits. I was always eating the wrong foods. I kept thinking I was too old to lose weight, so I never really bothered." Now that Eileen has reached her Goal Weight, her arthritis has improved so much that she rarely has any pains.

our 'By Mail' service. With Weight Watchers By Mail we will send you easy-to-follow material, similar to that used in Meetings, as well as information on all our products. There is also a Helpline manned by fully trained consultants who will answer any queries. If you would like further details phone our By Mail office on 091 296 2200.

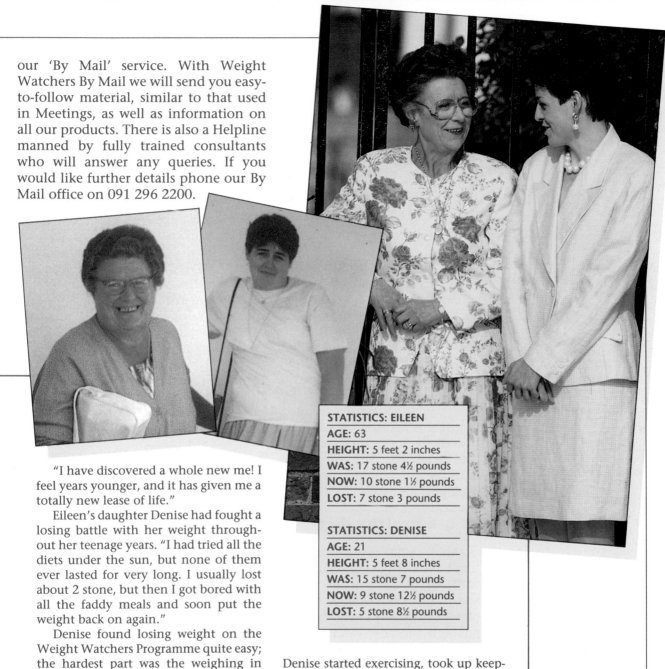

STATISTICS: EILEEN	
AGE: 63	
HEIGHT: 5 feet 2 inches	
WAS: 17 stone 4½ pounds	
NOW: 10 stone 1½ pounds	
LOST: 7 stone 3 pounds	

STATISTICS: DENISE	
AGE: 21	
HEIGHT: 5 feet 8 inches	
WAS: 15 stone 7 pounds	
NOW: 9 stone 12½ pounds	
LOST: 5 stone 8½ pounds	

"I have discovered a whole new me! I feel years younger, and it has given me a totally new lease of life."

Eileen's daughter Denise had fought a losing battle with her weight throughout her teenage years. "I had tried all the diets under the sun, but none of them ever lasted for very long. I usually lost about 2 stone, but then I got bored with all the faddy meals and soon put the weight back on again."

Denise found losing weight on the Weight Watchers Programme quite easy; the hardest part was the weighing in every week. "It is so difficult to come to terms with just how heavy you have become." However, she soon got over that hurdle and went from a size 24 to a trim size 12.

As well as changing her eating habits, Denise started exercising, took up keep-fit classes and swimming, and bought an exercise bike. Her main goal in life now is to stay in shape. "I'm determined to keep my figure, after working so hard to achieve my goal. I never want to go back to how I was."

The good news is that with Weight Watchers you can continue to eat most of the foods you really enjoy, in moderation, as part of a balanced healthy eating plan. It is no good just cutting down and eating less. This will leave you feeling hungry, hard done by and more likely to succumb to temptation, and may initiate a vicious circle of overeating and starving yourself. This only leads to disappointment and failure, not permanent weight loss.

What we offer you is a healthy alternative: a change of eating habits and a new balanced diet to last a lifetime. Remember that you are what you eat, and good nutrition is fundamental to good health. You need to get the balance right so that you eat a variety of foods that provide all the essential nutrients needed for your health and well-being. Our flexible Programme enables you to do just this because, as you will discover, we divide foods into six main groups, and every day you eat foods from each of the different groups to get the balance right. It's easy.

So what is a healthy diet?

Theories about what constitutes a healthy diet have changed dramatically in the last twenty years. Now all nutritionists and health experts agree that a healthy diet is one that is low in fat and sugar, and high in carbohydrates and fibre. The Weight Watchers Programme reflects the latest nutritional thinking and governmental guidelines.

To lose weight, you have to learn to take in fewer calories than your body uses in the form of energy. Exercise burns up some calories and if you combine this with a healthy eating plan, it will speed up your weight loss, but it takes a huge amount of energy to lose just one pound of body fat. As Professor Arnold Bender, the nutritional consultant to Weight Watchers, points out: 'Each pound contains over 3,500 calories, and therefore you'd have to run, jog or walk for many hours a day to get rid of just one pound. So the only real way to lose surplus weight is to reduce energy intake.'

On the Weight Watchers Programme you are encouraged to eat foods that provide all the nutrients recommended by the Government's COMA Report on Dietary Reference Values. This report laid down guidelines for healthy eating and nutrition, and specified the suggested maximum and minimum levels for daily intake of various nutrients.

COMA Report recommendations

The Report recommends that if you are to enjoy good health you must change your diet in the following ways:

● Reduce the amount of saturated fat – mostly animal fat – to 15 per cent of your total food energy intake

● Reduce all fat intake – saturated and polyunsaturated – to less than 35 per cent of your total energy intake

● Cut down on the amount of salt you use

● Eat less sugar. Replace fatty and sugary foods with high-fibre cereals and starchy unrefined carbohydrates

● Limit your alcohol intake

The Weight Watchers Programme meets all these requirements and will help to re-educate you and your family into a new healthier way of eating, which will not only help you lose weight but will also improve your general health and well-being.

Get the balance right

If you are eating fewer calories than you did in the past, it is more important than ever that your diet is finely balanced so that you get sufficient nutrients to maintain good health. Many slimming diets work by restricting your calorie intake but they do not achieve a nutritional balance. However, our Programme has been worked out by nutritionists to create a nutritionally balanced weight-reducing plan, with food you will enjoy. On our diet:

● You do not have to skip or substitute meals. On the contrary you must eat regular meals, so you reduce the chance of feeling hungry

● You can still enjoy the occasional snack or treat. No food is absolutely forbidden, although some foods should be eaten less often and in limited amounts

● You can eat as many fresh vegetables as you like, with the exception of starchy ones, such as broad beans, peas, potatoes, parsnips, sweetcorn, sweet potatoes and water chestnuts, which come from a different food group

● You can have the pleasure of eating real food. You do not replace meals with 'diet bars' and 'diet drinks'. You just eat normal everyday food that you and your family will enjoy

Healthy eating for you . . . and your family

The Weight Watchers Programme has divided the foods you eat into six different groups. These are as follows:

● Proteins
● Fats
● Milk and dairy produce

Foodfax: A healthy diet

Nutritionists agree that a healthy diet consists of eating:
● A variety of foods – for a balanced diet
● Less fat – to reduce the risk of obesity and heart disease
● Less salt – to reduce the risk of high blood pressure
● More fibre – to maintain bowel regularity and improve the digestive system
● Less sugar – to maximise nutrient intake and prevent tooth decay

● Fruit
● Vegetables
● Carbohydrates (Bread Selections)

Every day you need to eat a variety of foods taken from all these groups to achieve a balanced diet which will help you to reach your target weight and stay there in the future.

Protein – the body's building blocks

Protein is essential for building and repairing body tissues, organs and muscles. The following foods are all good sources of protein:

● Meat, poultry and fish
● Milk *, eggs and cheese (* included in Milk Selections)
● Pulses*, beans*, cereals* and nuts (*included in Carbohydrate (Bread) Selections)

Some foods, such as red meat, hard cheeses and nuts, are excellent sources of protein but they are relatively high in fat; you should restrict your intake to reduce your level of blood cholesterol. Thus it is better to opt for white meat like chicken, and white fish, rather than red meat, as they are lower in fat and calories. If you are a vegetarian you can get all the protein you need from lentils, beans, nuts, eggs, cheese and dairy produce. Eggs are high in cholesterol and for this reason you should eat no more than a maximum of seven a week.

Fats – a concentrated energy source

Fat has become a dirty word in our society and most people eat too much of it. Fats are high in calories and, if eaten in large quantities over a long period of time, a potential health risk. They are the hidden element in many of the processed foods we eat – like crisps, ice cream, mayonnaise, salad dressings, pastry, biscuits, cakes and chocolate. Because they are used in cooking and the processing of so many foods, you may not be aware of how much oil and fat you eat.

However, some fats are essential for your health and you should not cut them completely out of your diet. With this in mind, we ask you to select some fats every day as part of your balanced eating plan. You can choose from foods such as the following:

● Avocados and olives
● Vegetable oil and salad dressings made with polyunsaturated fats
● Low-fat spreads
● Nuts

Like everything else, fats can still be enjoyed – but in moderation. Eating too much saturated fat (animal fats in meat and dairy produce) not only leads to a weight problem, but also increases the cholesterol in your bloodstream, and this builds up inside your arteries and heart. This may eventually lead to blocked arteries and cause a heart attack. However, unsaturated fats will not raise your cholesterol level and will help to build and repair cells in the body. These fats are found in foods such as:

● Vegetable oils, especially sunflower, corn and soya
● Some brands of margarine
● Nuts and oily fish, e.g. herring and mackerel

Milk and dairy produce – vital for your health

Milk, cheese and yogurt are all good sources of protein and calcium, all important for building strong bones and teeth. Unfortunately, most dairy products tend to be high in fat, so you should switch to low-fat versions, like skimmed milk, low-fat yogurt, cottage cheese and low-fat cheeses. Foods such as cream, butter, full-fat cheeses and cream cheese should be eaten sparingly only as an occasional treat. You can try one of the low-fat spread alternatives to butter – some brands are excellent and have a good flavour. Instead of topping fruit desserts with a spoonful of cream, try using a low-fat natural yogurt as a more healthy alternative with a little artificial sweetener and vanilla essence.

Fruit and vegetables – Nature's gifts

Bursting with vitamins and minerals, which are essential for promoting good health, fruit and vegetables are two separate food groups (Selections) on the Weight Watchers Programme. They are an important source of fibre, which will add bulk to your diet and help you to

CINDY WITHERIDGE

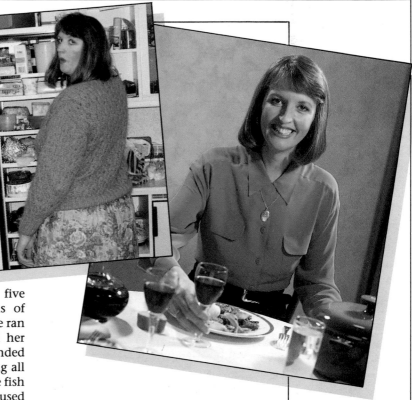

STATISTICS: CINDY
AGE: 41
HEIGHT: 5 feet 11 inches
WAS: 15 stone 12¾ pounds
NOW: 11 stone 4 pounds
LOST: 4 stone 8¾ pounds

Cindy had been overweight for five years, and had tried many forms of dieting before Weight Watchers. She ran a guest house and used to eat all her meals on the run, so usually she ended up having one big meal and picking all day. Cindy's main temptations were fish and chips, cakes and gâteaux. She used to finish any food that could not be served to guests. "It was terrible, I used to hide by the fridge eating broken bits of pavlova dipped in a bowl of cream!"

Her decision to join Weight Watchers came when she was serving at a wedding. She was trying to squeeze through with a tray, and a guest said, "Watch out – here comes the sumo wrestler!" Once on the Programme, Cindy did not find it difficult at all to change her eating habits. "You can eat normal, everyday foods. Nothing is bad – you fit it into the Programme. I used to eat mainly fish and chicken with a limited amount of red meat and fill up on vegetables.".

After losing nearly 5 stone and staying that way for 14 months, Cindy feels totally in control of her eating habits. She eats the same foods as she did on the Programme, but has larger portions. She can even feel happy about putting on a pound or two, as she knows she can take it off again. She is presently training to be a Leader, and says about the Weight Watchers Programme:"It's excellent and it works. You don't have to go shopping for faddy foods – you eat the same as the family and not rabbit food!"

Cindy's family are delighted with her new image. "My children are now happy to be seen out with me, and my husband says he has a new wife." Her family has also benefited from Cindy's change of eating habits. "They eat far more healthily; less fat, skimmed or semi-skimmed milk, more vegetables and regular meals."

Cindy succeeded through sheer determination, encouraged by her Leader and group chats. "We all help each other." It certainly worked for her.

feel full – a useful slimming aid. Fibre itself is indigestible and moves through the digestive tract to clear away body wastes.

On the Weight Watchers Programme you can eat a variety of fruit and vegetables. To get the maximum nutritional benefit from them, it is better to eat them raw rather than cooked if possible. This is because some vitamins, notably the B-group and vitamin C, are water-soluble and can be reduced by cooking. There are some fruit and vegetables which have to be cooked, and for advice on the best way of cooking these, turn to page 60. Fruit and vegetables add variety to your meals, making them more interesting. Vegetables have a particularly important role to play as many are virtually unlimited on the

CAROL WEATHERLEY

Carol Weatherley had tried nearly every diet possible before she discovered Weight Watchers. "My fiancé spent pounds on the new diets," she recalls, "but they never really worked."

She made the decision to try Weight Watchers when she was on holiday in the South of France. "I looked like a beached whale in a swimsuit; and I had no nice evening wear to go out in as all my clothes were too small."

On the Weight Watchers Programme, Carol lost nearly 5 stone and changed her eating habits and her life. "The Weight Watchers Programme is so easy to follow. You are allowed a little of everything. The support and friendliness of the Members is a boost, and you get great ideas from them. I am a lot healthier now and my eating habits are much better than they used to be."

Carol now eats a really varied diet with plenty of fresh fruit and vegetables as well as carbohydrates and protein foods. This is how she managed to lose weight, and now keeps it off and maintains her new slimline shape. Her hardest struggle was cutting out chocolate and sweet things, but now she can control her eating, and still enjoy these foods as occasional treats. She says: "I have had so many compliments, which I never had when I was fat. I go out a lot more than I did. I used to just sit in a corner and hide myself away. I am more confident and outgoing and I feel good. People can't get over how much weight I have lost. I don't think they thought I would do it. But that made me persevere all the more to prove them wrong." And how wrong they were!

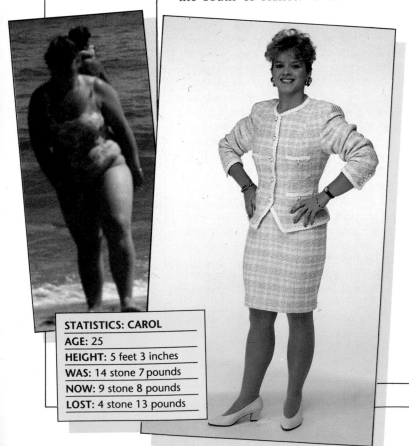

STATISTICS: CAROL	
AGE:	25
HEIGHT:	5 feet 3 inches
WAS:	14 stone 7 pounds
NOW:	9 stone 8 pounds
LOST:	4 stone 13 pounds

Programme. (with the exception of starchy ones).

You might think that fruit is also unlimited, but because it contains more calories than vegetables, there are restrictions on how much you should eat in a single day.

Carbohydrates (Bread Selections)

To our experienced Members, this food group is known as 'Bread Selections'. It includes bread, pasta, rice, beans, lentils, whole-grain cereals and starchy vegetables such as potatoes and peas. Cereals are a useful all-purpose food which, in addition to carbohydrate, will supply you with many essential nutrients: protein, fibre, vitamins and minerals. Whole-grain products, such as bread made with 100 per cent stoneground wholemeal flour, brown rice, whole-wheat pasta and whole-grain muesli, are higher in fibre and are more nutritionally valuable than their processed alternatives. Fibre is very important in your diet because it maintains bowel regularity and reduces the risk of colon cancer.

Foods from this carbohydrate group should make up a large part of your diet. They will provide you with energy as they are converted by your body into glucose and glycogen to fuel your muscles, brain and nervous system. Carbohydrates are mainly starches but they also come in the form of sugar, especially in fruit and milk.

Starch and sugars are the biggest sources of carbohydrates in most people's diets. Sugar and many other refined carbohydrates are virtually empty calories from a nutritional point of view, and contain little or no goodness. They are rapidly converted into glucose and absorbed into the bloodstream in quick bursts.

Unrefined carbohydrates are metabolized into glucose more slowly and released into the blood in a slower, steadier stream, providing you with a more sustained long-term supply of energy. On the Weight Watchers Programme, we suggest that you replace some of the fatty foods in your diet with unrefined carbohydrates. Use them to keep your energy levels topped up.

What are Selections?

We ensure that you have a completely nutritionally balanced diet by dividing all the foods you eat into groups. In this way, you can get the right number of calories to lose weight, as well as all the nutrients you need. Using this unique system, foods are categorized within the different groups already described: Carbohydrates (Bread Selections), Fats, Fruit, Milk, Protein and Vegetables. Each portion of food with its serving size in each food group is one Selection. On the following pages, you will see visual examples of Selections.

Each day women should eat 4 Carbohydrate (Bread) Selections, 3 Fat Selections, 3 Fruit Selections, 2 Milk Selections, 5 Protein Selections and 3 Vegetable Selections. This is the equivalent of approximately 1200 calories per day.

Each day men should eat 6 Carbohydrate (Bread), 4 Fat, 4 Fruit, 2 Milk, 7 Protein and 3 Vegetable Selections. Young people should follow the men's recommended food intake and add an extra ½ pint/300ml skimmed milk daily.

In addition to these Selections, you can have up to 100 extra calories of foods of your choice, which we call 'Optional Calories'.

Milk Selections...
at a glance

Milk is an important source of nutrients in your diet, and we recommend that everyone following our Programme should have a minimum of 2 Milk Selections each day (see the diet rules and guidelines for the special 14-day Programme on pages 118/119). Men and young people must have additional Selections. Pictured below are the foods that represent one Milk Selection.

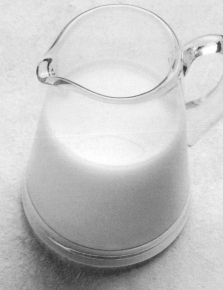

½ pint/300ml skimmed milk

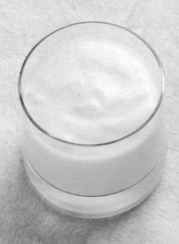

5fl oz/150ml low-fat natural yogurt

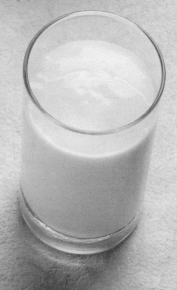

1oz/30g low-fat dried milk

½ pint/300ml buttermilk

Fat Selections... at a glance

When you're on a diet, it is important to cut down on the amount of fat you eat, but you still need to have some fat each day to maintain good health. The foods featured here represent one Fat Selection. You can see that by using low-fat alternatives you can make the most of your Fat Selections. We recommend that women following our Programme should have 3 Fat Selections each day, and men and young people should have 4 Fat Selections each day. Beware of tempting 'nibbles' like nuts and olives which contain hidden fats.

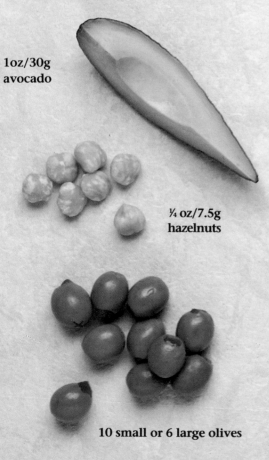

1oz/30g avocado

¼ oz/7.5g hazelnuts

10 small or 6 large olives

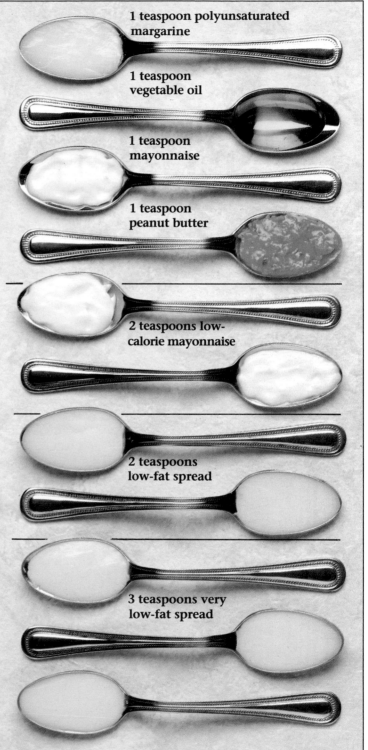

1 teaspoon polyunsaturated margarine

1 teaspoon vegetable oil

1 teaspoon mayonnaise

1 teaspoon peanut butter

2 teaspoons low-calorie mayonnaise

2 teaspoons low-fat spread

3 teaspoons very low-fat spread

What can I eat?

Protein Selections... at a glance

All the foods photographed here represent one Protein Selection. Women should eat 5 Protein Selections each day, and men and young people should eat 7 Protein Selections each day. Please note that the foods which are marked with an asterisk on this page are all 'limited' because they are relatively high in saturated fat and cholesterol, and therefore you should restrict your weekly intake of them. You may eat a maximum of 7 eggs a week and 14oz/420g of red meat and hard cheese. Vegetarians can ensure that they get adequate Protein Selections from foods such as cheese, eggs, tofu and beans.

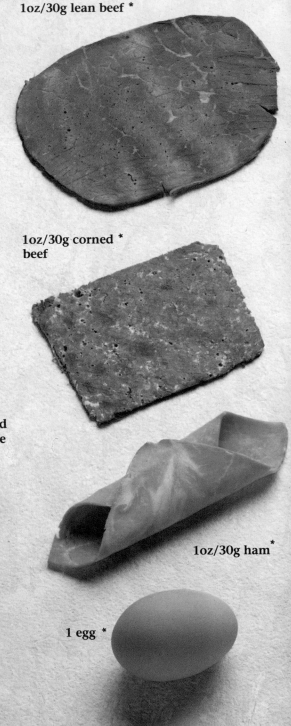

1oz/30g lean beef *

1oz/30g corned * beef

1oz/30g ham *

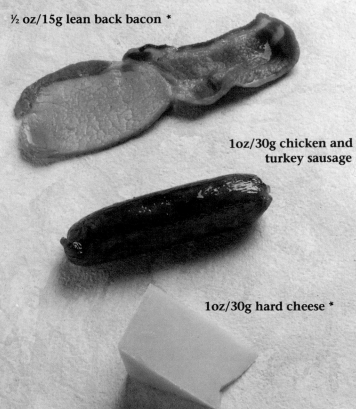

½ oz/15g lean back bacon *

1oz/30g chicken and turkey sausage

1oz/30g hard cheese *

1 egg *

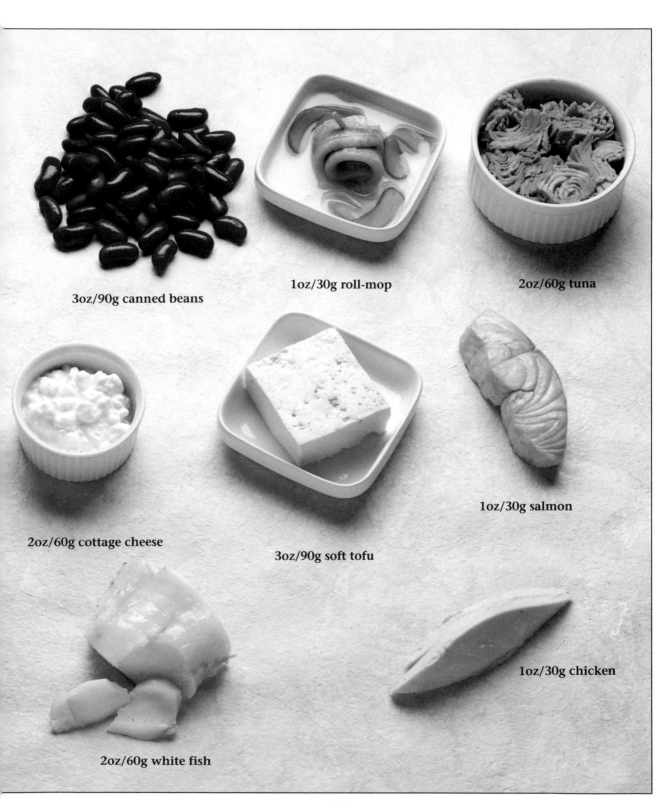

3oz/90g canned beans

1oz/30g roll-mop

2oz/60g tuna

2oz/60g cottage cheese

3oz/90g soft tofu

1oz/30g salmon

2oz/60g white fish

1oz/30g chicken

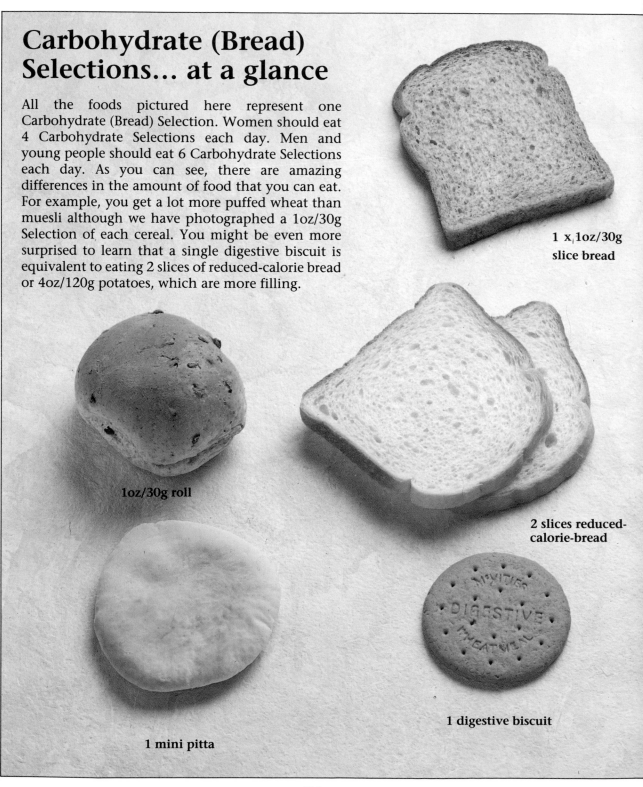

Carbohydrate (Bread) Selections... at a glance

All the foods pictured here represent one Carbohydrate (Bread) Selection. Women should eat 4 Carbohydrate Selections each day. Men and young people should eat 6 Carbohydrate Selections each day. As you can see, there are amazing differences in the amount of food that you can eat. For example, you get a lot more puffed wheat than muesli although we have photographed a 1oz/30g Selection of each cereal. You might be even more surprised to learn that a single digestive biscuit is equivalent to eating 2 slices of reduced-calorie bread or 4oz/120g potatoes, which are more filling.

1 x 1oz/30g slice bread

1oz/30g roll

2 slices reduced-calorie-bread

1 digestive biscuit

1 mini pitta

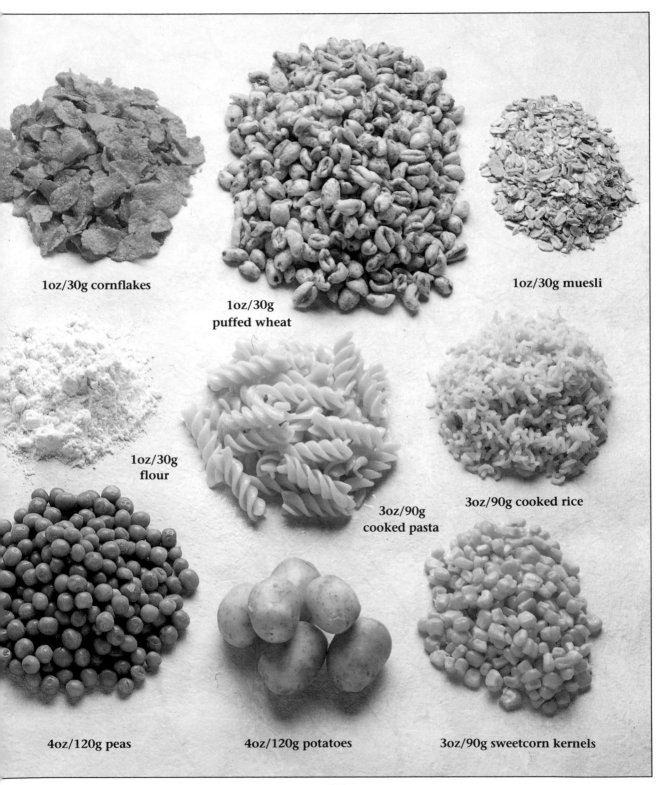

1oz/30g cornflakes

1oz/30g
puffed wheat

1oz/30g muesli

1oz/30g
flour

3oz/90g
cooked pasta

3oz/90g cooked rice

4oz/120g peas

4oz/120g potatoes

3oz/90g sweetcorn kernels

Fruit Selections... at a glance

You might think that there is nothing healthier and more slimming than filling up on fruit when you are on a diet. However, on our Programme fruit is limited. Women should eat 3 Fruit Selections each day. Men and young people should eat 4 Fruit Selections each day. Even dried fruit and fresh fruit juices fall within this category and you should control the amounts you consume. Everything pictured here represents one Fruit Selection.

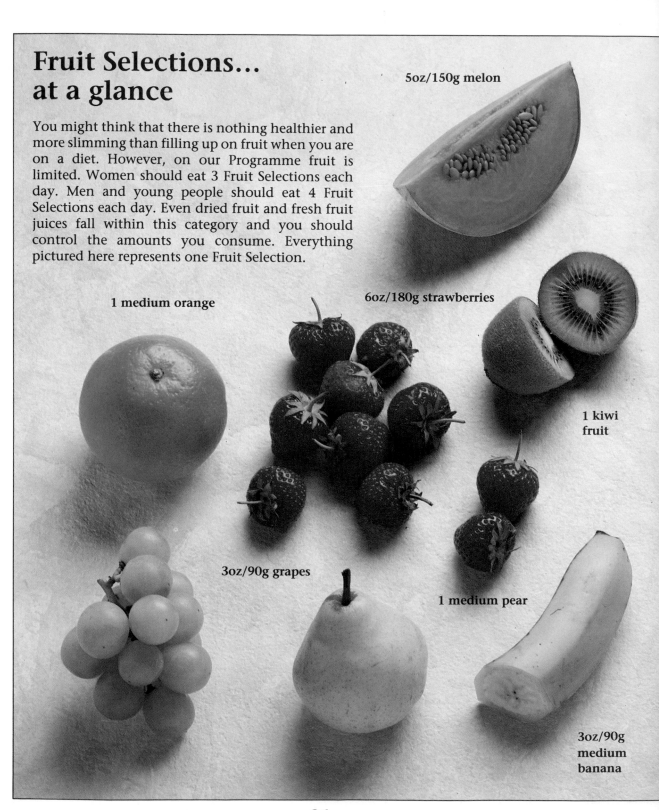

5oz/150g melon

1 medium orange

6oz/180g strawberries

1 kiwi fruit

3oz/90g grapes

1 medium pear

3oz/90g medium banana

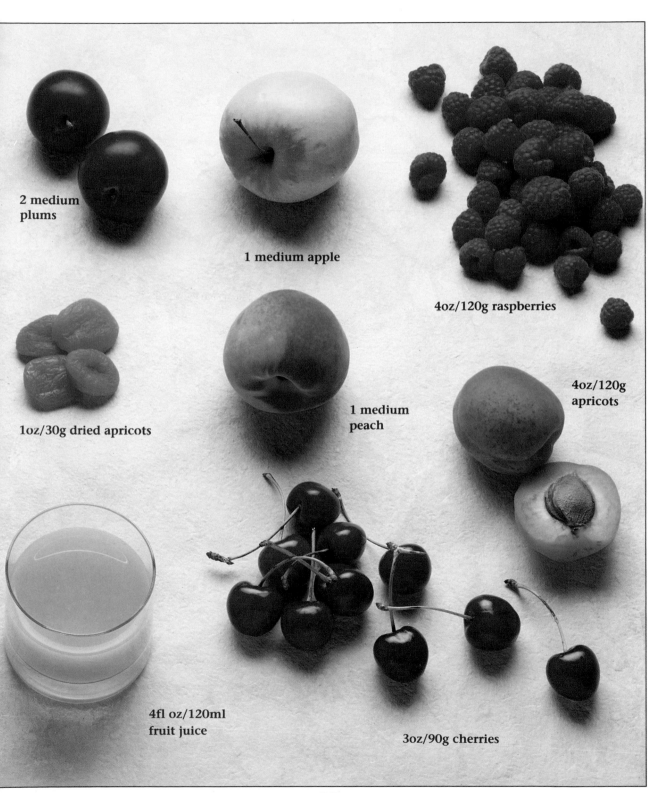

2 medium
plums

1 medium apple

4oz/120g raspberries

1oz/30g dried apricots

1 medium
peach

4oz/120g
apricots

4fl oz/120ml
fruit juice

3oz/90g cherries

Vegetable Selections... at a glance

All the vegetables featured here are shown in 3oz/90g portions, which represents one Vegetable Selection. As you must eat at least 9oz/270g of vegetables each day (3 Selections), they are a great way of bulking out your diet and making it more interesting and versatile. Remember that starchy vegetables, e.g. parsnips, peas, potatoes, sweetcorn, sweet potatoes and water chestnuts, are not counted as Vegetable Selections. You will find these in the Carbohydrate (Bread) Selections.

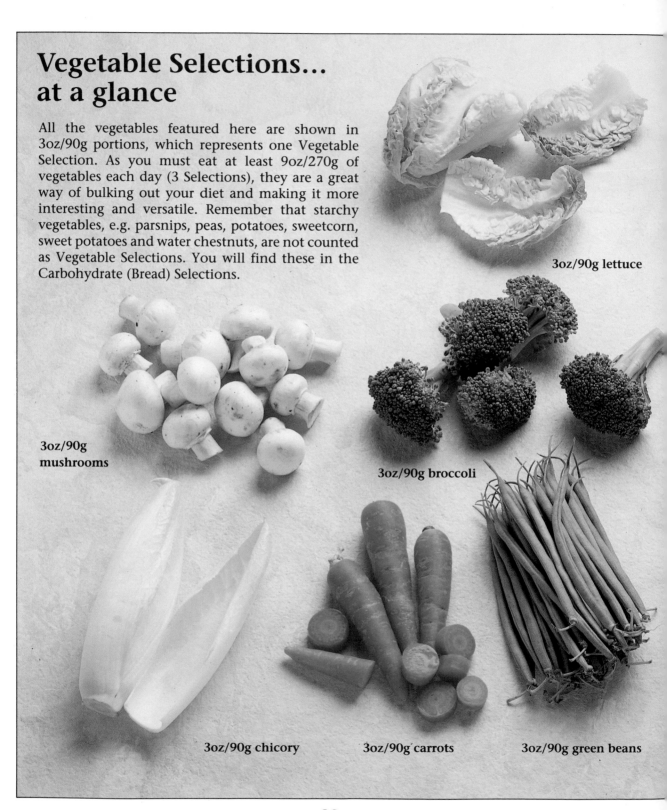

3oz/90g lettuce

3oz/90g mushrooms

3oz/90g broccoli

3oz/90g chicory

3oz/90g carrots

3oz/90g green beans

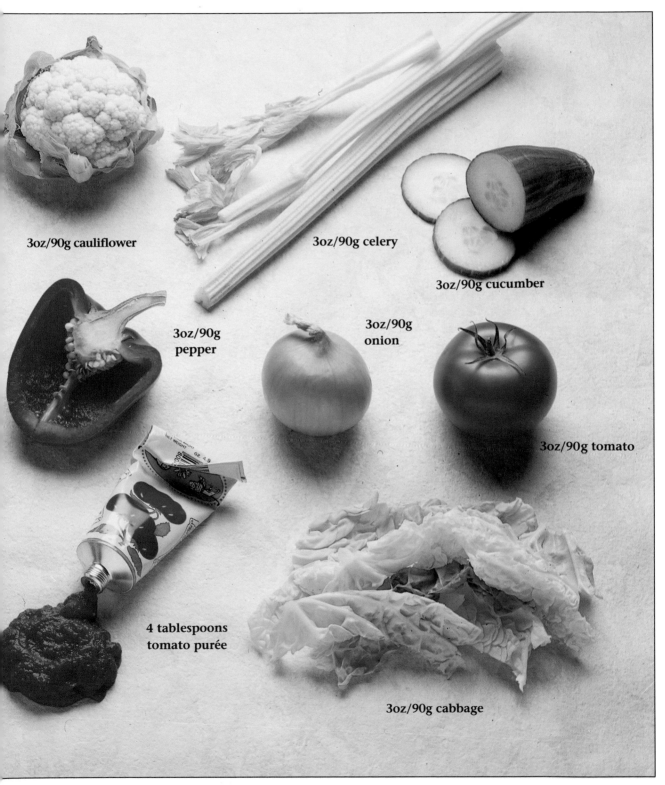

3oz/90g cauliflower

3oz/90g celery

3oz/90g cucumber

3oz/90g pepper

3oz/90g onion

3oz/90g tomato

4 tablespoons tomato purée

3oz/90g cabbage

Optional Calories... at a glance

With the Weight Watchers Programme you do not normally have to worry about calorie counting as foods are shown as Selections. However, in addition to your Selections, you are allowed (if you wish) 100 Optional Calories each day. This allowance is the same for women, men and young people. You may 'spend' your Optional Calories on foods that do not obviously fit into a Selection group or on any convenience food that only shows calories per serving on the packaging. Or simply use your Optional Calories to treat yourself to a favourite food. You can also save up your Optional Calories and have a more substantial treat every few days or at the weekend.

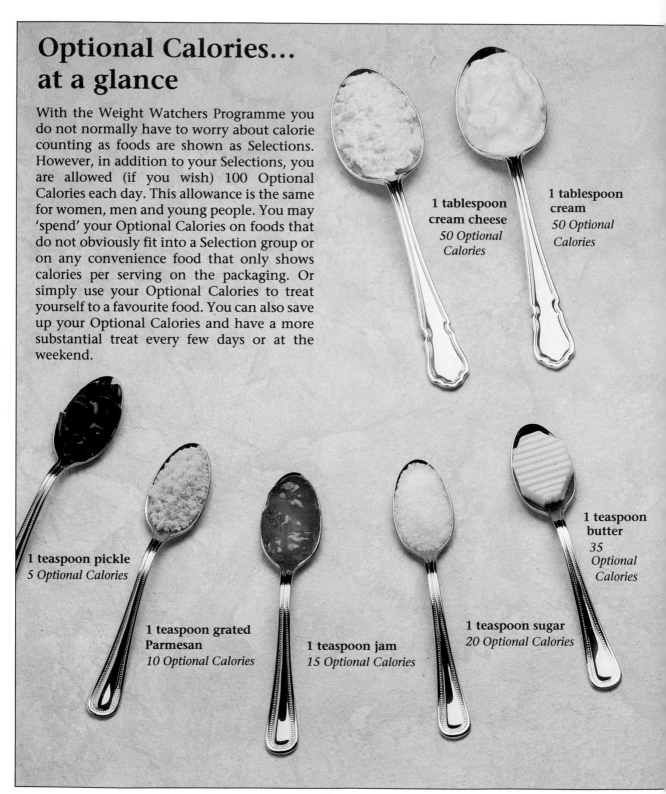

1 tablespoon cream cheese
50 Optional Calories

1 tablespoon cream
50 Optional Calories

1 teaspoon pickle
5 Optional Calories

1 teaspoon grated Parmesan
10 Optional Calories

1 teaspoon jam
15 Optional Calories

1 teaspoon sugar
20 Optional Calories

1 teaspoon butter
35 Optional Calories

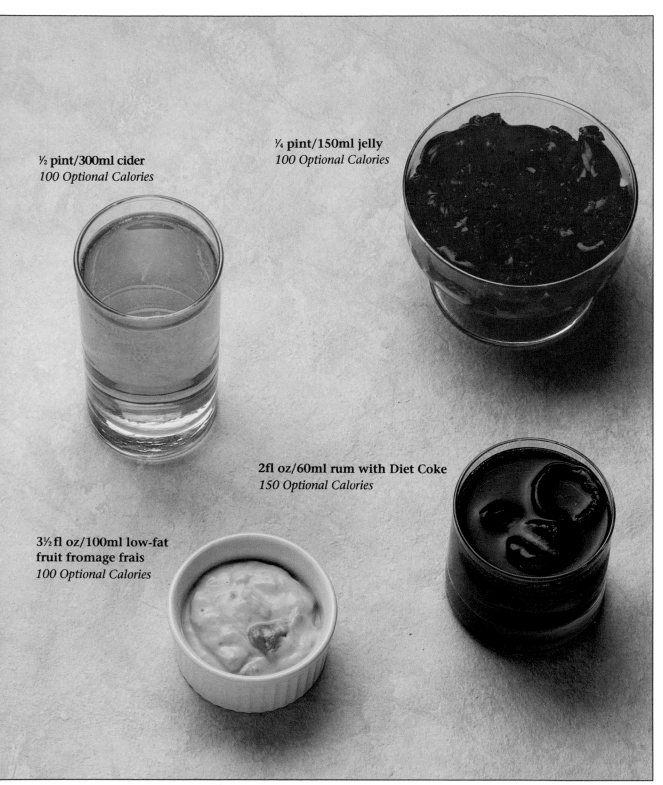

½ pint/300ml cider
100 Optional Calories

¼ pint/150ml jelly
100 Optional Calories

2fl oz/60ml rum with Diet Coke
150 Optional Calories

3½ fl oz/100ml low-fat
fruit fromage frais
100 Optional Calories

Combination Foods...
at a glance

Combination Foods contain Selections taken from one or more food groups and extra Optional Calories too. If you are keeping an eye on what you eat and how many Selections and calories each food contains, you should be aware of these foods and count your Selections carefully. All the foods shown here are examples of Combination Foods.

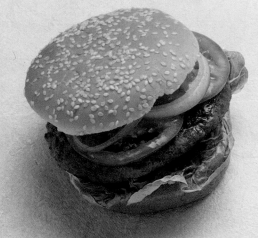

1 beefburger with bun
Selections: 2 Bread, 1½ Protein

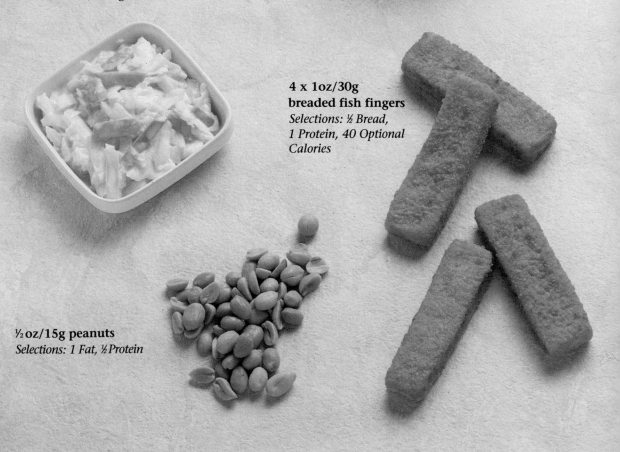

3oz/90g coleslaw
Selections: 2 Fat, 1 Vegetable

**4 x 1oz/30g
breaded fish fingers**
*Selections: ½ Bread,
1 Protein, 40 Optional
Calories*

½ oz/15g peanuts
Selections: 1 Fat, ½ Protein

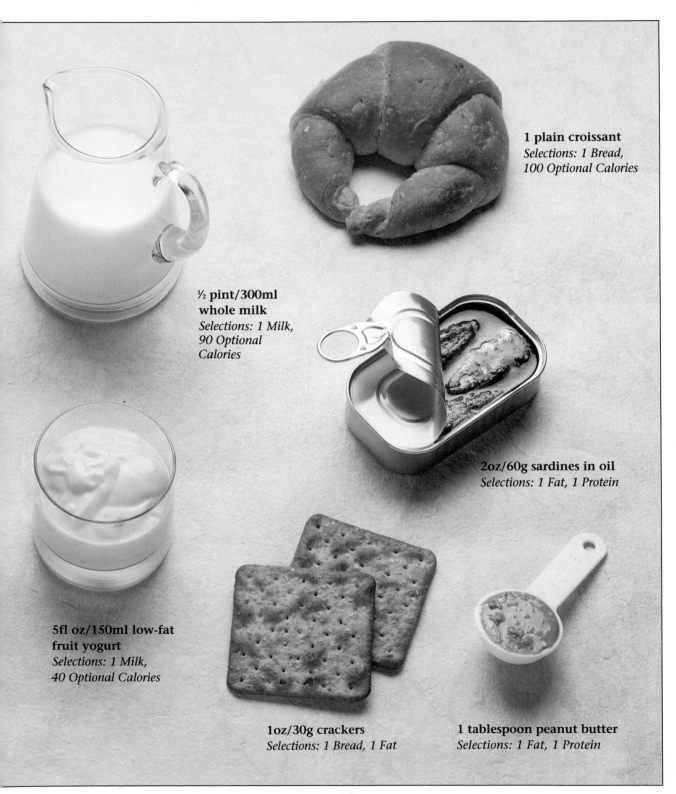

1 plain croissant
Selections: 1 Bread,
100 Optional Calories

½ pint/300ml
whole milk
Selections: 1 Milk,
90 Optional
Calories

2oz/60g sardines in oil
Selections: 1 Fat, 1 Protein

5fl oz/150ml low-fat
fruit yogurt
Selections: 1 Milk,
40 Optional Calories

1oz/30g crackers
Selections: 1 Bread, 1 Fat

1 tablespoon peanut butter
Selections: 1 Fat, 1 Protein

Convenience foods... at a glance

We all tend to eat convenience foods, but many of them contain hidden fats and sugars. It is worth remembering that some are less healthy than others. For example, beans on toast is higher in protein and fibre and contains less fat than a pork pie or a small chocolate bar. However, beans are relatively high in sugar, so, if you are keeping an eye on what you eat, it might be a good idea to opt for one of the special reduced-calorie, low-sugar products. If you know the nutritional content of these foods you can include them in your Selections (see page 29) or use your Optional Calories to enjoy them.

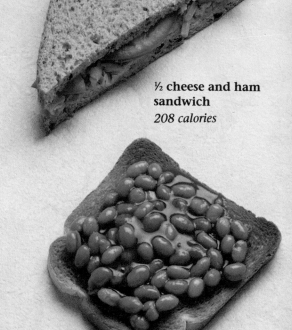

½ cheese and ham sandwich
208 calories

5.3oz/150g beans on toast
210 calories

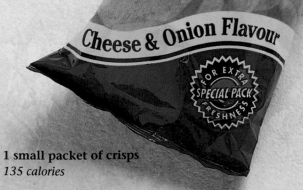

1 small packet of crisps
135 calories

1 spring roll
240 calories

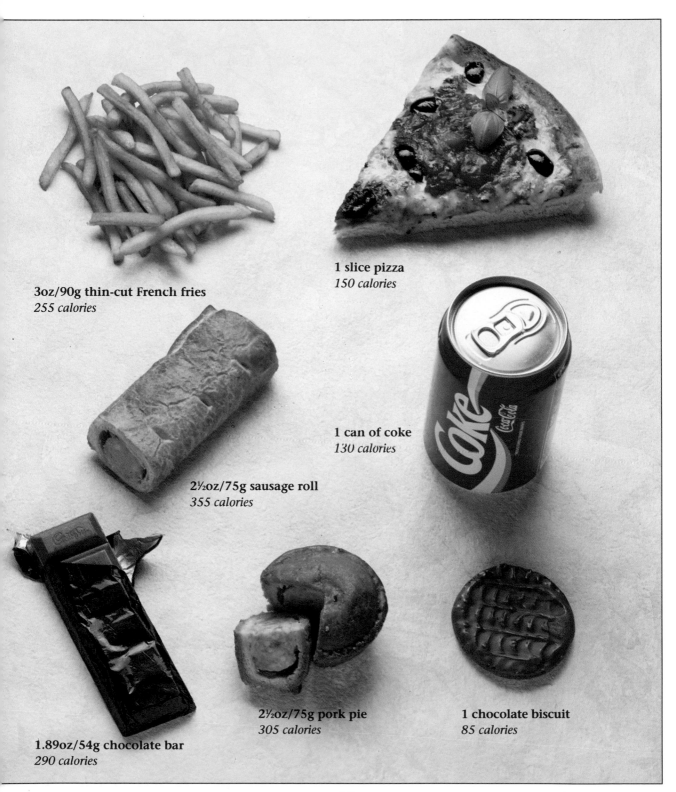

3oz/90g thin-cut French fries
255 calories

1 slice pizza
150 calories

2½oz/75g sausage roll
355 calories

1 can of coke
130 calories

1.89oz/54g chocolate bar
290 calories

2½oz/75g pork pie
305 calories

1 chocolate biscuit
85 calories

Hidden calories... at a glance

Many everyday foods contain hidden calories; even a small portion can yield a lot of unwanted calories and little in the way of nutritional goodness. On these pages, we have featured some of the foods of which you should be wary. They may taste delicious but they can represent danger to the person who is trying to lose weight. Be aware of the hidden calories in some foods; you can still enjoy then occasionally, but in moderation.

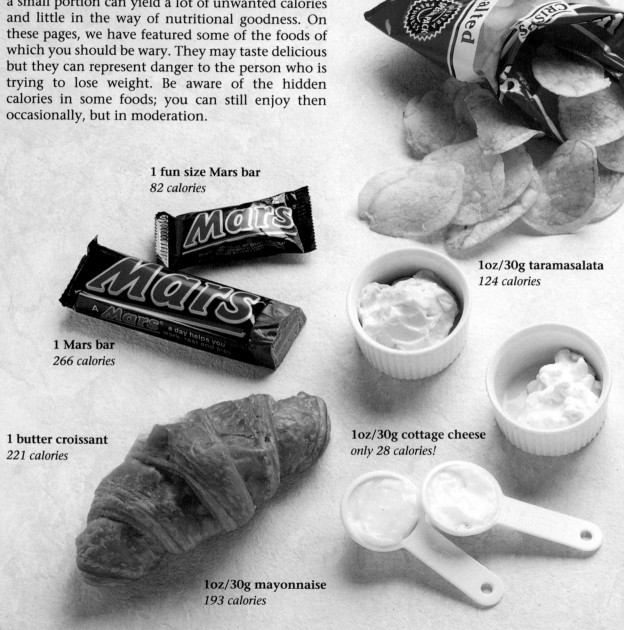

1 small packet of crisps
135 calories

1 fun size Mars bar
82 calories

1 Mars bar
266 calories

1 butter croissant
221 calories

1oz/30g taramasalata
124 calories

1oz/30g cottage cheese
only 28 calories!

1oz/30g mayonnaise
193 calories

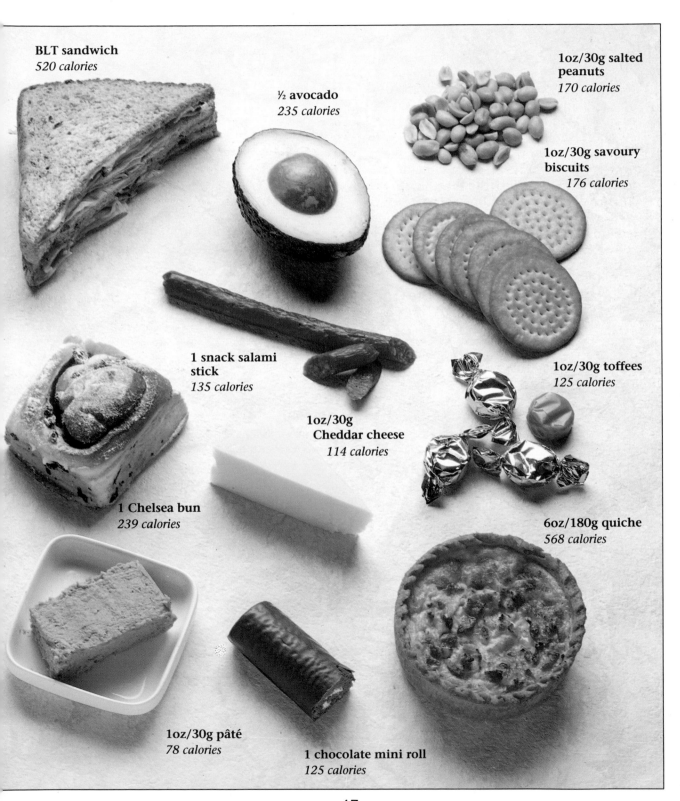

BLT sandwich
520 calories

½ avocado
235 calories

1oz/30g salted peanuts
170 calories

1oz/30g savoury biscuits
176 calories

1 snack salami stick
135 calories

1oz/30g Cheddar cheese
114 calories

1oz/30g toffees
125 calories

1 Chelsea bun
239 calories

6oz/180g quiche
568 calories

1oz/30g pâté
78 calories

1 chocolate mini roll
125 calories

Treat yourself!

We know that everybody enjoys a little treat occasionally, and with these calorie-counted foods you can treat yourself without ruining your diet. You may be surprised to discover how many, or indeed how few, calories there are in some of your favourite foods. For example, just five squares of whole nut chocolate amounts to 200 calories, whereas for only 100 calories you can treat yourself to a large bowl of fresh strawberries – and some cream!

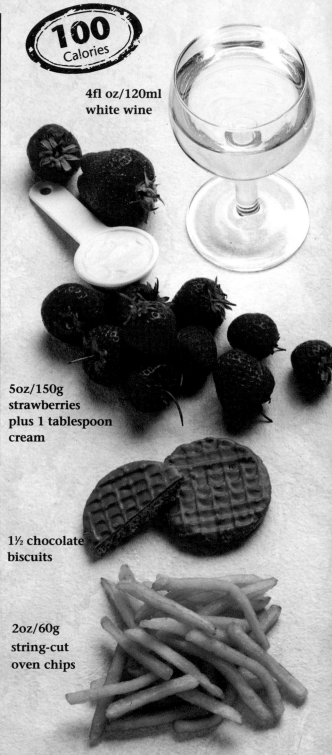

100 Calories

4fl oz/120ml white wine

5oz/150g strawberries plus 1 tablespoon cream

1½ chocolate biscuits

2oz/60g string-cut oven chips

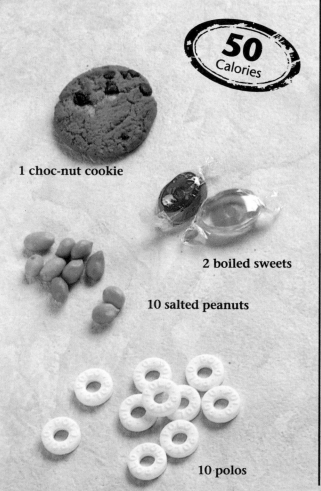

50 Calories

1 choc-nut cookie

2 boiled sweets

10 salted peanuts

10 polos

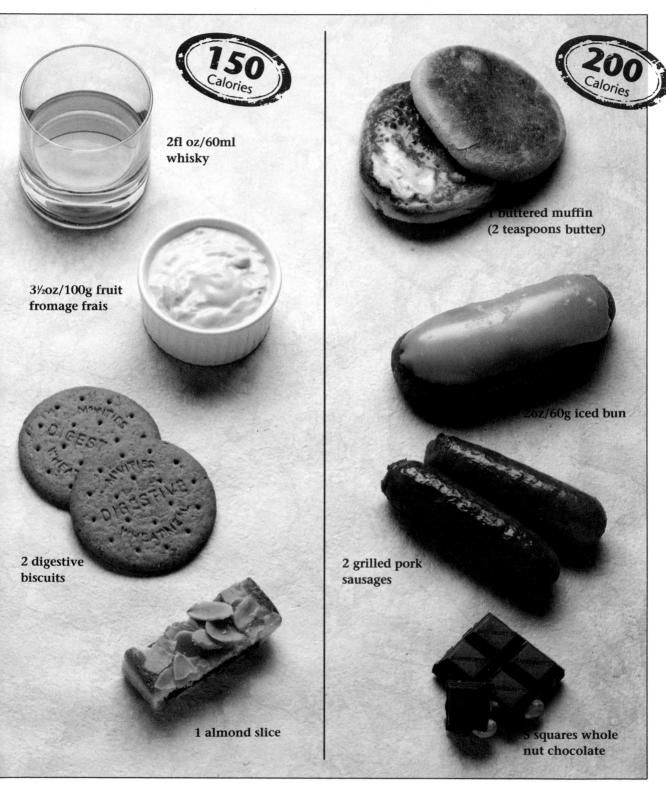

150 Calories

2fl oz/60ml whisky

3½oz/100g fruit fromage frais

2 digestive biscuits

1 almond slice

200 Calories

1 buttered muffin (2 teaspoons butter)

2oz/60g iced bun

2 grilled pork sausages

3 squares whole nut chocolate

VEGETARIANS

The Weight Watchers Programme caters for vegetarians and non-vegetarians alike. We work together with the Vegetarian Society to prepare meals that are suitable for our vegetarian Members. The 14-day Programme (see page 118) includes a menu plan specially designed for vegetarians.

You can choose Selections from the same Food Lists by opting for vegetarian choices. For example, you can still have all the Carbohydrate (Bread), Fat, Fruit, Milk and Vegetable Selections, while on the Protein List, you can choose from eggs, beans, nuts, lentils, tofu, low-fat cheese and textured vegetable protein.

In this way you can continue to enjoy well-balanced vegetarian meals while you lose weight. Try adding variety to your diet by experimenting with new vegetables and cooking them in different ways. With the exception of the starchy vegetables (broad beans, parsnips, peas, potatoes, sweet potato, sweetcorn and water chestnuts), most

---

Shoppingfax: If you are vegetarian
When you go out shopping, bear in mind the following guidelines from the Vegetarian Society:
● All cheese must be vegetarian cheese
● All eggs must be free-range – not farm-fresh or barn eggs
● The mayonnaise you buy must be egg-free
● All margarines and low-fat spreads must be suitable for vegetarians

---

Vegetable soup

This is a useful standby when you are feeling hungry between meals or want to add bulk to a main meal. You do not have to stick to the suggested vegetables in the recipe; you can try adding or substituting green beans, celery, leeks, peppers or swede. This soup is very low in calories, but you can transform it into a more filling light meal by adding more Selections; for example, by sprinkling some grated cheese on top and serving it with reduced-calorie or wholemeal bread. Alternatively, you can add 1oz/30g dried milk powder to make the soup more creamy. The following recipe makes two servings. If wished, you can double the quantities given and freeze the additional portions individually.

VEGETABLE SOUP

1 medium onion, finely chopped
2 garlic cloves, crushed
1 medium courgette, thinly sliced
1 medium carrot, chopped
1 medium tomato, skinned and chopped
1 teaspoon chopped fresh parsley
pinch of dried basil
pinch of ground black pepper
¾ pint/450ml vegetable stock (made with 1 cube)

1 Put all the ingredients in a saucepan, cover and simmer for about 20 minutes until the vegetables are tender.
2 You can serve the soup like this, or, if you like a smoother less chunky result, you can purée the mixture, or purée half the soup and stir in the remaining chunky vegetables.
3 Return to the pan to reheat and then serve.

JOYCE CASWELL

Joyce Caswell made the decision to join Weight Watchers when she looked in a shop mirror and imagined herself in a few years as 'fat and forty'. She thought she looked matronly and old, even though she was only in her mid-thirties. That was nine years ago, and since then Joyce has lost over 2½ stone and become a Tutor for Weight Watchers.

Joyce had a very busy life working long hours, and consequently used to be a 'snacky eater'. After her evening meal Joyce would watch TV and eat more sandwiches, biscuits or crisps.

She joined Weight Watchers and says, "I needed someone to tell me I could do it, and give me the encouragement I needed."

Joyce is a vegetarian but she had no problems with the Weight Watchers Programme. She started eating regular meals, three a day, for the first time ever. She loves cooking and found that it was easy to use the Programme and adapt many recipes to a vegetarian way of eating.

STATISTICS: JOYCE	
AGE: 44	
HEIGHT: 5 feet 5 inches	
WAS: 12 stone 2 pounds	
NOW: 9 stone 8½ pounds	
LOST: 2 stone 7½ pounds	

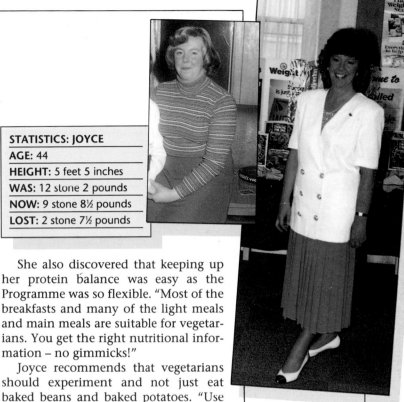

She also discovered that keeping up her protein balance was easy as the Programme was so flexible. "Most of the breakfasts and many of the light meals and main meals are suitable for vegetarians. You get the right nutritional information – no gimmicks!"

Joyce recommends that vegetarians should experiment and not just eat baked beans and baked potatoes. "Use some imagination." Because many vegetables are virtually unlimited, you can still eat a lot and need never feel hungry."

are virtually unlimited and you can eat as many as you wish: as an accompaniment to meals and in between meals as snacks and nibbles. In fact, eating extra vegetables is a good way of bulking out meals and keeping hunger pangs at bay.

Make protein a priority

To add protein to vegetables, you can try the following:

● Make a crunchy nut topping for savoury bean and vegetable bakes and casseroles. But beware! Use the nuts sparingly as they are high in fat

● Sprinkle a little grated cheese over steamed vegetables and gratins

● Top baked jacket potatoes with low-fat cheese or baked beans

● Mix canned beans into salads

● Add beans and lentils to chunky vegetable soups and stews

● Thread tofu on to vegetable kebabs

● Stir some cooked or canned beans and nuts into stir-fried vegetable dishes

● Add a beaten egg, herbs and grated cheese to hot drained pasta and cook quickly, to make a 'carbonara' sauce

● Sprinkle grated cheese over vegetable risottos and rice dishes

PREGNANCY & BREASTFEEDING

The old saying goes that 'you are what you eat' and this is particularly true when you are pregnant. Your baby needs good food to grow, to develop and to build up tissues, and so, to a great extent, he/she *is* what you eat. If you do not eat a balanced diet during pregnancy you could deprive your baby of the nutrients needed for normal growth and development. When you are pregnant, your nutritional requirements are high.

You can see from all this that pregnancy is not a good time for embarking on a weight loss programme unless there is a very good medical reason for doing so and you are under the supervision of your doctor. However, it should not be an excuse to overeat and stuff yourself with nutritionally worthless calories. Being seriously overweight carries its own risks during pregnancy and delivery, including developing high blood pressure, backache and having a more difficult labour.

Good nutrition, not weight loss, should be your aim since a sensible rate of weight gain is important for the health of your baby. If you follow our general guidelines for a healthy diet and eat a wide range of foods from the different food groups you should avoid putting on excess weight during your pregnancy, which is a problem for many women. Pregnancy is a time for eating well and gaining an adequate amount of weight.

How much should I gain?

During pregnancy, it is quality, not quantity, that counts, and, contrary to popular belief, you do *not* have to eat significantly more calories than usual each day. During the first three months you will need only an extra 150 calories per day, rising to 350 calories per day in the last six months. When you consider that two more slices of wholemeal bread a day equals approximately 150 calories, you can see that it is not a lot of extra food. Eating for two really is a myth.

For many years, doctors believed that it was beneficial to restrict your weight gain during pregnancy as they considered that excessive weight gain was linked to a high incidence of toxaemia. However, research shows that women on poor diets who restrict their weight are more likely to suffer pregnancy and labour complications and give birth to low-birthweight babies.

Mothers on good, nutritious diets tend to gain about 28 pounds on average and give birth to bigger, healthier, stronger babies. A child's birthweight usually increases proportionately to the mother's weight gain during pregnancy. So do not attempt to restrict

Where the weight goes

Weight gain	in pounds
Baby's birth weight	7.5
Placenta	1.5
Amniotic fluid	2
Enlarged uterus	2
Enlarged breasts	1.5
Increased blood volume	4
Increased body fluids & fat	9.5
Total weight gain:	28

LYNN SIVELL

Lynn Sivell didn't have a weight problem until she left school. "I was a skinny child, quite a tomboy, and I was quite good at sport. It was when I left school and stopped playing sport that I started to put on weight. I was always about a stone overweight and on a diet. I would lose a few pounds, and then put them back on again."

When Lynn got pregnant with her first child, she gained 4 stone. After her daughter was born, she carried an extra two stone for years – until she joined Weight Watchers. Meanwhile, Lynn tried all sorts of diets and gimmicks, even slimming pills, but she never got down to her ideal weight.

She first went to Weight Watchers in 1977, and although she lost 16 pounds, she didn't reach her Goal Weight. Lynn says, "I thought I would do the rest on my own but it didn't work out, so I went back to Weight Watchers again and lost the last 12 pounds. My husband used to be a professional footballer and played for Ipswich Town. When Ipswich won the FA Cup in May 1978, it was a double celebration because that's when I reached my Goal Weight."

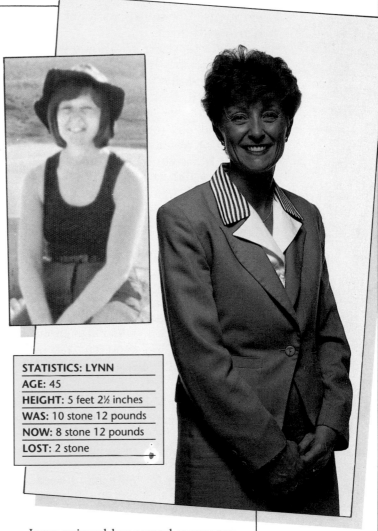

STATISTICS: LYNN	
AGE:	45
HEIGHT:	5 feet 2½ inches
WAS:	10 stone 12 pounds
NOW:	8 stone 12 pounds
LOST:	2 stone

Lynn became a Leader later that year, and in January 1979 she became pregnant. She carried on taking her Meetings until the day before she went into labour. "During my pregnancy, I was very sensible about what I ate. I followed the basic Programme, and ate extra protein and skimmed milk, and more fruit and vegetables. It was a really healthy balanced diet. I only gained 21 pounds in total during my pregnancy, and gave birth to a healthy little boy of 8 pounds 7 ounces. I was back at my Goal Weight two weeks later, and I have kept the weight off ever since."

Lynn enjoyed her second pregnancy more than her first one, which was very traumatic. "When I had Adam, I was so healthy, fit and well. I had learned enough from Weight Watchers to eat a nutritionally balanced diet and avoid putting on excessive weight. The birth was easier and I felt so much better."

Lynn has been a Weight Watchers Leader for fifteen years and she is now a National Trainer, still helping other people to lose weight and take control of their lives.

your intake of nutritious foods – your baby needs them.

So how much weight should you gain and where does it all go? Most doctors recommend that you gain 10 pounds in the first 20 weeks, and approximately one pound per week thereafter until birth, making a total of 28 to 30 pounds. You may wonder how all this extra weight is accounted for – after all your baby probably weighs only about six-and-a-half to eight-and-a-half pounds at birth. The excess weight is not all fat. Look at the table on page 52 to see how it is calculated.

Women who are overweight when they conceive may be better off gaining less as long as they receive all the essential nutrients for their baby's growth and development. You can check whether you are gaining superfluous weight by measuring your upper thighs regularly; however much weight you gain throughout your pregnancy your

TRACEY STINGEMORE

Tracey's weight problem started after her marriage. She tried all sorts of diets, none of which worked, before joining Weight Watchers and losing most of her excess weight. However, then she became pregnant. Her new-found healthy eating habits stood her in good stead, and as soon as she was able, after the baby was born, she went back to Meetings until she reached her Goal Weight.

Throughout her pregnancy, Tracey continued to eat a good selection of healthy foods, and this helped to prevent her from putting on excessive weight. "I lost most of my extra weight at Weight Watchers shortly before I became pregnant. As soon as my baby was born, I went back determined to reach my Goal Weight, and I did!" Now that she knows how to eat a really balanced diet, she can maintain her slim shape with ease, and educate her family into eating the healthy way.

"Weight Watchers worked for me because the Food Plan is everyday food: food that the whole family can eat and enjoy. There are plenty of good recipes to choose from, and healthy eating is very important to me now."

Losing weight has really boosted Tracey's confidence, and she now lives life to the full. "When I was overweight, I didn't like to go out for meals because I felt people were looking at me, thinking: 'She's fat – she doesn't need to eat.' Now I can wear the clothes I like and everyone comments on the way I look. They can't believe how much I eat and still stay slim."

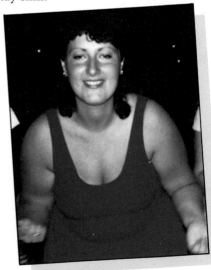

thigh measurements should stay roughly the same.

Many women worry needlessly that if they do not restrict their weight, they will have a large baby or a more painful delivery, but this could not be further from the truth. Your labour problems probably decrease, rather than increase, as the size of the baby increases. Women who give birth to smaller babies often tend to have longer, more difficult labours as their uterine contractions are weaker if they have eaten a poor diet.

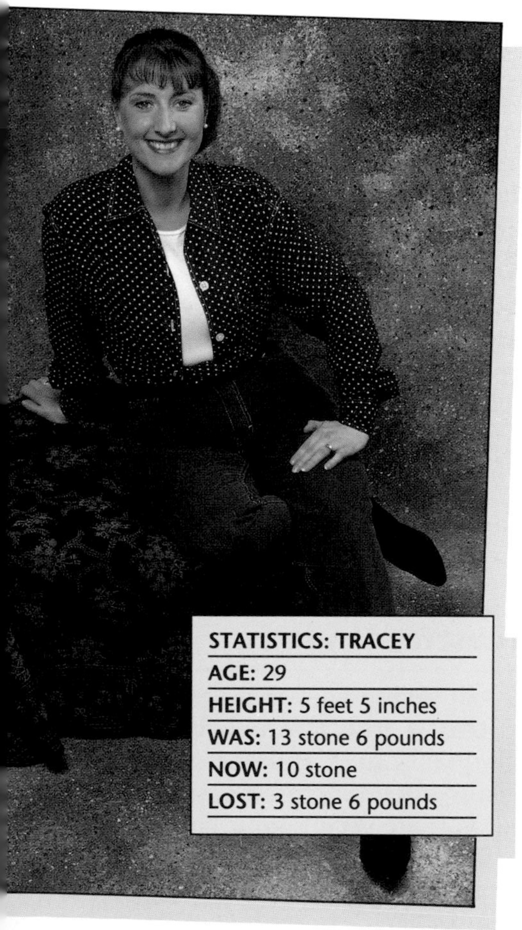

What should I eat?

There are no special foods for pregnancy that you *must* eat, but you should aim to have a healthy varied diet with the emphasis on high quality nutritious food. Always choose natural wholesome alternatives to sugary, refined and processed foods, whenever possible, and avoid eating too many fats.

Basic rules

- Cut out sugar or, at least, cut down
- Avoid over-refined convenience foods that contain artificial additives
- Cut down on saturated fats, especially butter and cream
- Drink and cook with skimmed milk and eat low-fat natural yogurt every day; these supply essential vitamins and minerals as well as protein
- Eat more fibre, especially whole-grain cereals, beans, fresh fruit and vegetables
- Get adequate protein from meat, fish, poultry, cheese, grains, eggs and vegetables

You can see that these dietary requirements are very similar to those of the Weight Watchers Programme. If you are worried about destroying your successful weight loss to date or regaining excess weight, talk to your doctor and, if you are attending Meetings, your Weight Watchers Leader. They will be able to advise you on the best course of action and put your mind at rest.

Weight Watchers pregnancy plan

Weight Watchers has developed a special plan to help you get the nutri-

STATISTICS: TRACEY

AGE: 29

HEIGHT: 5 feet 5 inches

WAS: 13 stone 6 pounds

NOW: 10 stone

LOST: 3 stone 6 pounds

tional goodness that you and your baby need. You will need your doctor's approval to follow this plan; your local Leader will be able to give you more details. For safety's sake, we advise that you do the following:

- Avoid alcohol
- Reduce your intake of caffeine, and sugar substitutes
- Eat iron-rich foods such as lean meat and dried fruit, and foods that are high in folic acid like dark green leafy vegetables, broccoli and oranges
- Do not eat unpasteurized soft cheeses
- Do not eat raw egg or eggs that are not hard-boiled
- Do not eat mayonnaise that contains raw egg
- Do not eat liver or liver products – ask your doctor's advice on this

Avoiding common problems

To help you feel better throughout your pregnancy we advise that you take note of the following tips:

- To deal with nausea, poor appetite and vomiting, eat smaller, more frequent meals and 'graze' your way through the day. Eat bland, simple foods – not rich and spicy ones. This will help you avoid heartburn too in the later months
- If constipation is a problem, drink plenty of water and select foods that are high in fibre, especially whole-grain bread and cereals, fruit and vegetables
- If you cannot drink milk due to allergies or intolerances, make sure that you get your protein and calcium requirements from other foods such as cheese, yogurt, sardines, salmon and broccoli. Or ask your doctor for a calcium supplement

Exercise during pregnancy

Pregnancy is not the best time to begin an exercise programme, other than at a supervised prenatal class. However, if you have been exercising regularly before your pregnancy – at least three times a week – you may be able to continue exercising at a moderate pace provided that you follow these guidelines:

- Avoid jerky, bouncing movements
- If you feel any unusual muscle strain, stop immediately
- Warm up prior to exercise and end your session by cooling down and stretching gently
- Drink water before, during and after exercise to prevent dehydration
- Use gentle toning exercises to firm up calves, thighs, hips and upper arms and prevent superfluous weight gain

If you are unsure about what is safe to do, ask your doctor or midwife for advice, or enrol at a special prenatal exercise class.

Breastfeeding

The old saying goes that 'breast is best' and this is true if you have sufficient high-quality milk and don't experience any nursing problems. If you can breastfeed, you are giving your baby the best possible start in life, providing all the nutrients needed for growth and development as well as antibodies to protect against allergy and infection.

The milk you produce is specially formulated to nourish your baby and provide the right nutrients in the correct proportions. Breastfeeding presents you with a nutritional challenge, as you must eat a really healthy diet with adequate nutrients and calories – at a time when you are probably longing to regain your pre-pregnancy figure.

The quality of your milk

You need to eat nutrient-rich food, especially meat, chicken, fish, eggs, cheese, yogurt, milk and whole-grain cereals, fresh fruit and vegetables. If you eat sensibly and avoid over-refined convenience foods and too much fat and sugar, breastfeeding can help you to regain your figure.

The quality of your milk depends on the raw materials you use. Your total calorie requirement will be higher now than during pregnancy, and you will need approximately 350 extra calories a day. Your own body stores will be mobilized to meet some of the nutritional requirements for producing milk. If you try to cut down on calories to lose weight, your milk supply will be affected.

In the early weeks it is usually better to eat the more easily digested protein foods, such as yogurt and low-fat cheeses, skimmed milk, chicken and fish. You also need vegetables, fruit, whole-grain cereals, polyunsaturated vegetable fats and plenty of fluid, especially water and fruit juice. You may find that some foods you eat disagree with your baby, especially rich, spicy dishes, leeks, onions and garlic.

Regaining your figure

During your pregnancy, fat was stored by your body in preparation for lacta-

> **Important**
>
> We do not recommend that you eat soft cheeses (particularly unpasteurized cheese) or eggs (unless they are hard-boiled) nor any products containing raw eggs, e.g. mayonnaise. We also recommend that you should not eat liver or liver products, including pâté and sausage, whilst you are nursing.

tion. This fat will be used up gradually in your daily milk production. Even though you cannot cut down too much on the amount of food you eat and you have to maintain a high-quality nutritious diet, you will eventually lose weight and regain your figure, especially if you exercise regularly.

The same rule applies as during your pregnancy: it is quality, not quantity, that counts. As long as you eat a healthy diet and cut out – or keep to a minimum – fattening foods like cakes, pastries, chocolate, cream, sugar and biscuits, you should get all the nutrients you need and shed some excess weight.

We have a special Food Plan for nursing mothers which you can follow, with your doctor's approval. The demands of nursing your baby are so great that it is critical for you to concentrate on proper nutrition before weight loss. You will need extra nutrients if you are to provide an adequate milk supply. As you begin to introduce your baby to solid foods, you can start to cut down slowly on the extra food you are eating. However, whilst you are nursing your baby, it is not appropriate to return to your pre-pregnancy weight by cutting down on essential nutrients.

CHILDREN

Just like you, your children need to eat good, nutritious food if they are to grow healthy and strong and are to avoid putting on excessive weight. However, for many children, processed convenience foods, which are high in fat and sugar, have become the norm, and some rarely eat any fresh fruit, vegetables, whole-grain cereals or wholemeal bread. The odds are that you feed your children the sort of food you eat yourself, so by changing your diet to a more healthy one, you can protect their health too.

Feeding your baby

Good food habits start in early life. Introducing solid foods too early and feeding too many high-fat, sugary foods help to make children overweight. Babies need variety just as we do – fresh fruit, vegetables, yogurt, fish, chicken and cereals can all be whizzed up in different combinations in a blender.

Feeding your toddler

Toddler food is a step up from baby food. Toddlers don't like mushy, puréed foods – they're babyish! You can tempt them to eat a healthy diet by providing interesting-looking finger foods of fresh fruit and vegetables. They need milk and yogurt, wholemeal bread and sugar-free

cereals, protein foods such as meat, poultry, fish, eggs, cheese and beans. Give them fruit juice or water to drink rather than fizzy sugary drinks, and avoid sugar, sweets, crisps, chocolate, biscuits, cream and sugar-coated breakfast cereals.

It is important not to overfeed; give toddlers as much as they want and don't encourage them to clear the plate if they have had enough. Serving sizes will vary according to a child's mood, age, level of activity, appetite, growth rate, general state of health and even the climate.

Feeding your schoolchild

When children start school, it is more difficult to control their diet as they will come into contact with other children and eat out at parties and with friends. What matters most is the food you serve up at home every day. This becomes the norm, the basis of their future health and food preferences. Every mealtime you should try to provide:

● Protein food, e.g. meat, fish, poultry, eggs, cheese, milk, beans and yogurt
● Fresh fruit and vegetables
● Unrefined carbohydrates, e.g. wholemeal bread, pasta, rice, wholewheat breakfast cereals, potatoes

Breakfast is particularly important as twelve to fourteen hours have passed since your children last ate the previous evening. Always provide a nutritious breakfast, e.g. muesli or unsweetened cereal, bread or toast, poached, boiled or scrambled egg, unsweetened fruit juice. You can offer cooked foods such as grilled sausages or bacon but it is not necessary. Avoid bran-based cereals,

Healthy baby foods
● Sugarless baby cereals
● Sugar-free fruit juices with added vitamin C
● Fresh fruit purées
● Fresh vegetable purées
● Sugarless rusks
● Vegetable juices
● Puréed chicken or fish with vegetables

which are too high in fibre for young children.

School lunches

Your child may benefit from cooked school meals, and most schools and local authorities have improved the nutritional quality of the meals on offer in recent years. There is more emphasis on high-fibre, low-fat dishes served with fresh fruit, vegetables and salads.

However, many children take packed lunches and these must be planned carefully to ensure variety and nutritional balance. Children soon get bored with the same old sandwich fillings every day. Many children's lunch boxes are still packed with sweets, crisps, chocolate bars and processed foods, but it doesn't take a lot of time, imagination or money to offer interesting alternatives.

Teas and suppers

If children eat a healthy breakfast and a nutritious cooked or packed lunch, they will not necessarily need a large evening meal. Obviously, a balanced meal of meat/fish and vegetables is very healthy, but most children prefer a high tea – a substantial snack-type meal which can be prepared quickly and easily when they arrive home from school. Offer nutritious snacks like beans on toast, baked potatoes, eggs (poached, boiled or scrambled), soup, omelettes or fish fingers. Try and serve some salad or vegetables with the meal and finish with some fresh fruit, a yogurt, fruit salad or jelly.

The overweight child

A fat child is rarely a happy child. Being overweight can mean torment and misery as children are notoriously unkind to their peers. Games lessons can be embarrassing and they can often suffer unkind taunts. For your children's health and happiness, try to ensure that they don't become overweight. A sensible diet will keep their weight within a healthy range for their height, age and build. If you think that your child is significantly overweight talk to your doctor or health visitor.

Healthy weight guidelines

● Cut down on sugar – add fresh or dried fruit to cereal for sweetness

● Don't fry foods – grilling is healthier and does not add unwanted calories and fat to a dish. Jacket or boiled potatoes are healthier than chips; grilled fish beats fried fish; and eggs are better boiled or poached rather than fried

● Use skimmed milk for older children – it provides all the protein, calcium and vitamins of full-fat milk

● Offer healthy snacks – of vegetables, fresh fruit, juices, wholewheat biscuits, dried fruit; not sugary soft drinks, cakes, sweets, crisps and chocolate

● Ensure your child does not feel hungry – they may be tempted to snack on unhealthy foods. Bulk out meals with lots of fresh vegetables

● Make sure your child exercises – overweight children tend to lead sedentary lives, but any form of physical activity will help burn excess calories and tone up the body. Encourage your child to eat an early tea and then run about and play games afterwards, not settle down in front of the TV. Go to the swimming pool, for family walks and bike rides

With the Weight Watchers Programme you can cook lower-calorie versions of many of your favourite meals. It is not just the foods and the raw ingredients that are important but also the cooking methods you use.

Healthy cooking methods

These can affect your health and your shape. The ones we recommend are just as quick as, say, frying and boiling, yet they are more nutritious

● When cooking vegetables, it is better to steam them to guard against loss of nutrients, especially the water-soluble B and C vitamins which are partially destroyed by boiling and lost into the cooking water. If you must boil them, tip the prepared vegetables into boiling lightly salted water and boil very rapidly until just tender but still slightly crisp. However, steamed vegetables have more flavour and retain their goodness

● The best cooking methods for meat and poultry are grilling, baking and cooking in a casserole. Frying and roasting in fat add unwanted calories and destroy vitamins. Using quick cooking methods at high temperatures, e.g. grilling, helps to preserve nutrients

● In the case of fish, the best cooking methods are steaming, grilling and baking. An excellent way to cook cutlets and steaks is to wrap them in foil or greaseproof paper and bake in a moderate oven

● Stir-frying is another good way of cooking food very quickly. You cook thin strips or small chunks rapidly over a high heat, stirring in the minimum of oil. You can use this method for cooking vegetables, fish, seafood, chicken and

PENNY CARVOSSO

Penny Carvosso feels that she has gained a new lease of life since she lost 5 stone 1 pound with Weight Watchers. "No-one can possibly understand the total misery being fat envelops you in. I feel as though I have just escaped from a prison sentence, albeit self-imposed."

Being a Cordon Bleu cook and restaurateur did not help Penny's weight problem, which has been a constant one throughout her marriage, and especially after her two children were born. Over the years, Penny tried numerous diets but without success. "I must be the only person I know who always seemed to be on a diet. I thought I could do it my way! I have only been successful this time because finally I admitted to myself that I had to have help. I followed the Weight Watchers Programme to the letter. It worked for me because it's so flexible. I didn't feel as though I was dieting – it became a way of life."

The key to losing weight and staying slim is eating correctly, and for Penny it meant changing her basic diet and eating habits. "I now buy brown bread, skimmed milk and lots of fruit. We all eat more vegetables, and for breakfast I always have plain yogurt and orange

most lean cuts of meat such as sirloin.

Saving time and effort

Most of us don't want to spend long hours in the kitchen slaving over a hot stove if we can help it, especially when we're trying to lose weight. The less time you spend in the kitchen the better; this will help minimize temptation.

You can produce delicious and nutritious slimming meals with the

STATISTICS: PENNY
AGE: 44
HEIGHT: 5 feet 5 inches
WAS: 14 stone 2 pounds
NOW: 9 stone 1 pound
LOST: 5 stone 1 pounds

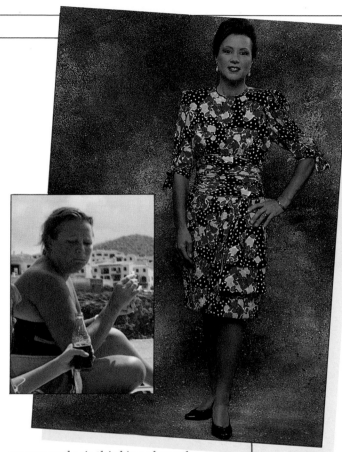

juice. I don't pick between meals anymore, and that's the biggest change."

Lunch is Penny's main meal of the day, when she enjoys a low-fat meal based on healthy eating. In fact, she is so impressed with Weight Watchers that she has introduced more slimming options on to her restaurants' menus.

Penny and her husband have an extremely busy lifestyle, owning a restaurant and wine bar in London, two hotels, and a restaurant in Menorca, but she has not had to make any compromises or changes to her life. "The best thing about Weight Watchers is that my life hasn't changed. At the end of the day I can't afford to change my lifestyle. I had to lose weight and keep the same lifestyle but eat a different way."

Penny's family has also benefited from her change of diet. "Hopefully my children will grow up accepting healthy eating as part of their life. I now serve fruit a great deal, and I notice how my plain yogurts disappear. It's nice that everyone else is thinking along the same healthy lines."

Penny has now won her personal battle and she is confident that, with her new healthy approach to eating, she can stay slim.

minimum of labour and time, especially if you grill and stir-fry foods quickly and make use of kitchen aids and equipment to cut down on preparation and cooking. Never be afraid of taking short-cuts and using gadgets when practical.

We have selected recipes which are relatively quick and easy to prepare and cook. This is especially important if you have a busy lifestyle combining a job with the demands of looking after your family and running a home. What you need is healthy fast food which is nutritious and low in calories, which will comply with our guidelines for healthy weight loss.

Adding variety to your diet

Many people perceive slimming food as being monotonous and boring, an endless round of undressed salads! However, on our 14-day Programme you will eat interesting, well-balanced meals.

You can add variety to your diet in many ways, especially with vegetables, which are unlimited. This means that you can eat as many as you like every day – with the exception of starchy vegetables such as potatoes, parsnips, sweetcorn, peas, broad beans, sweet potatoes and water chestnuts. Eating extra vegetables has many benefits including the following:

● They are a good way of bulking out meals

● They satisfy hunger between meals

● They are low in calories

● They provide essential vitamins and minerals

● They are a good source of fibre

You can eat vegetables raw in salads or as crudités (dipping sticks) with a low-calorie dip. You can eat them cooked: steamed, stir-fried or made into soups, casseroles, gratins and crunchy topped 'pies'. You can mix them with rice or pasta in a tasty low-fat sauce.

To prevent your diet becoming boring, choose a variety of different foods each day, raw and cooked, using different cooking methods and sauces to ring the changes. If you choose different foods from the various food groups at every meal, you will ensure that your meals are really varied and never dull.

Creating unusual salads

Don't just settle for some lettuce leaves, a tomato and some cucumber. Be more adventurous and experiment with different vegetables and low-calorie dressings to create some really unusual salads. Here are some ideas to try:

● Watercress, orange segments and chopped red onion in an orange vinaigrette dressing

● Grilled red, green and yellow peppers with crushed coriander seeds in a garlic-flavoured dressing

● Chicory, hazelnuts and green pepper in a whole-grain mustard dressing

● Shredded carrots, peanuts and herbs in a lemon vinaigrette dressing

● Cooked thin French beans in a warm vinaigrette dressing

● Drained canned beans, e.g. kidney beans, haricot beans or chick peas, mixed with tuna and sliced onion in a vinaigrette dressing

Cooking on a budget

You don't have to spend a fortune to lose weight. When shopping and planning your daily meals, bear in mind that 'expensive' does not necessarily mean 'best', from the point of view of nutrition and flavour. Cheaper chicken joints and economical fish fillets are just as nutritious as steak or salmon. You can cook them in numerous ways to produce interesting slimming meals for you and your family.

You can supplement more expensive sources of protein, such as meat and

Budget tips
● Buy seasonal fruit and vegetables when they are cheap and plentiful
● Make more use of rice, pasta and vegetables to bulk out meals and make a little meat or fish go a long way
● Make more use of eggs, cheese, beans etc.
● Use cheaper cuts of meat but remove all fat
● Use chicken wings, thighs and drumsticks rather than breast fillets

fish, with economical foods, such as eggs, low-fat cheese, skimmed milk, beans, pulses, seasonal vegetables and whole-grain cereals like wholemeal bread, rice and pasta, which are all rich in nutrients and relatively inexpensive.

Weighing and measuring food

When you start your diet you should weigh and measure all the food you eat so that you can be sure that you are getting the right amounts. This is particularly important during the early days when you are less familiar with portion control and are more likely to over-estimate permissible quantities. If you guess incorrectly and eat larger amounts than we suggest, you will lose weight more slowly; if you eat smaller amounts you may not be getting enough nutrients.

When you grow more accustomed to judging and recognising amounts easily, you need only weigh portions of food when you are uncertain of a precise measurement or when you are eating something new. Portion control is an important skill that will help you maintain your weight loss in future.

If you attend your local Weight Watchers Meeting, your Leader and fellow Members will give you tips on quick and easy measuring. However, if you do not already have some, you should invest in some accurate kitchen scales which will weigh very small quantities, a set of measuring spoons and a measuring jug.

Measuring tips

● Weigh in imperial (pounds, ounces, pints, fluid ounces) or metric (grams, kilogrammes, litres) measurements: do

> ### Cookingfax: Kitchen know-how
> ● Keep tempting foods out of sight and in sealed containers
> ● Don't cook more than you need so that you can avoid leftovers
> ● Don't pick at food and keep tasting it while you are cooking
> ● Don't finish up the leftovers so as not to 'waste them'
> ● When preparing food, put away any ingredients you do not intend to use in the larder or refrigerator as soon as you have measured out what you need. Don't leave them lying around on the work surface for you to pick at

not use both within the same recipe

● Always use level tablespoons or teaspoons unless a recipe calls for a heaped spoon, which can contain two to three times the recommended amount

● If your scales do not weigh less than 1oz/30g, then weigh that amount and divide into two for ½ oz/15g, or four for ¼ oz/ 7.5g

● Remember that 1 tablespoon is 15ml, and a teaspoon is 5ml, so you can measure small amounts of liquid with spoons rather than in a jug which may not record very low fluid measurements

Making your cooking more healthy

You can cook more healthy, slimming food by cutting down on fat and sugar. It's really very easy when you know how, and after a while it will become second nature to you to follow our guidelines. You will probably find that you do not enjoy fatty foods as much as you used to, and that even your taste for sweet things might recede a little.

How do I cut down on fat?

One of the first and most important things to learn when cooking the 'slim' way is how to reduce the fat content of everyday meals.

● **Grill instead of fry:** Many foods such as fish, chicken joints, chops, steak, sausages and bacon can be grilled without fat rather than fried in a pan. Place them on a rack over a grill pan so that any excess fat drips out of the food and can be discarded easily

● **Stir-fry instead of fry:** Vegetables can be quickly stir-fried with chicken, fish or meat cut into small chunks or strips in the minimum of oil

● **Always grill mince:** When making dishes using minced beef, e.g. chilli con carne, shepherds pie, spaghetti bolognese, do *not* add the mince to the sautéed onion and vegetables and cook in the oil. This only adds unwanted fat. Instead, grill the mince until the fat drips out, and then add the drained mince to the vegetables

● **Use less oil:** When cooking or stir-frying food, use only the tiniest amount of oil: two or three teaspoons will usually suffice. In salad dressings reduce

---

Slimfax: Quick conversions

When you measure foods as part of your weight loss plan remember these simple basic conversions for easy measuring:
● 1 level teaspoon = 5ml
● 1 level tablespoon = 15ml
● 1oz = 30g
● 1lb = 480g
● 1fl oz = 30ml
● ¼ pint = 5fl oz = 150ml
● ½ pint = 10fl oz = 300ml
● 1 pint = 20fl oz = 600ml

Healthfax: Eat more fibre
● Choose high-fibre breakfast cereals
● Eat more beans, peas and lentils
● Increase your daily vegetable intake
● Cook potatoes in their skins
● Choose wholemeal bread

---

the amount of oil used and add more lemon or orange juice, herb-flavoured vinegars, mustard, garlic or fresh herbs

● **Don't fry potatoes:** The best way to cook potatoes is to bake them in their skins so that they retain all their nutritional goodness. Serve with low-fat cheese or fromage frais instead of butter

● **Don't fry eggs:** Poach or boil them instead. Or make an omelette with the tiniest portion of low-fat spread

● **Forget about cream:** You don't have to cook with cream to make delicious sauces. Make white sauces with skimmed milk and cornflour. Instead of adding a small carton of cream to a savoury dish just before serving, create a creamy sauce by removing the pan from the heat and gently stirring in some low-fat natural yogurt or fromage frais

● **Use a non-stick pan:** It is possible to 'fry' food in the minimum of oil in a good quality non-stick frying pan. Wipe the pan with a minute quantity of oil or low-fat spread before cooking

● **Use a low-fat cheese:** Try the wide range of low-fat alternatives now available. (A real 'low-fat' cheese is one with fewer than 180 kcal per 100g.)

How do I cut down on sugar?

Most of us enjoy desserts and sweet dishes and it may be very hard to cut down on them. However, you can con-

VERITY KERRY

On a round-the-world trip, Verity Kerry put on 36 pounds during the seven months she spent travelling with husband Glyn. Verity literally ate her way round the world, but came back to reality with a bump when she landed at Heathrow. "I was fat and frumpy and none of my old clothes would go anywhere near me! I put on a happy front, but deep down I was becoming uncomfortable with my weight and that made me self-conscious. Every Monday I'd half-heartedly start another diet.

However, Verity wasn't shaken into action until a friend told her bluntly to stop complaining about her weight and do something."You're the only one who can!" This was just what Verity needed and she joined her local Weight Watchers Meeting. Weight Watchers' sensible approach to eating fuelled Verity's willpower, and in just 10 weeks she achieved her Goal Weight.

Verity was amazed at the large quantities she could eat on the Programme, and that she could still enjoy her favourite pasta dishes; it was just a case of adapting recipes to the low-fat Weight Watchers way. She threw away her frying pan and opted for grilling, baking or steaming instead.

Verity was losing between one-and-a half and two-and-a half pounds a week and finding it easy. "My only setback

STATISTICS: VERITY	
AGE: 27	
HEIGHT: 5 feet 4 inches	
WAS: 11 stone 9½ pounds	
NOW: 9 stone 1 pound	
LOST: 2 stone 8½ pounds	

was one week when I decided I no longer needed to weigh my food and put on a quarter of a pound."

Even now that Verity has reached her goal, she still wouldn't be without her food weighing scales. "I've completely changed my outlook on 'slimming'. I know now that it's a matter of being aware of what you're eating for life, not just for a few weeks. Food is no longer my enemy. I look forward to mealtimes because I've always got something delicious planned – and that stops me nibbling in between meals too."

tinue to eat these foods in moderation if you reduce their sugar content.

● **Use artificial sweetener:** In many desserts you can substitute this for sugar

● **Use fresh fruit as a natural flavouring:** Use it chopped or just the juice as a natural sweetening agent

● **Use dried fruit:** This can be used

sparingly to sweeten cakes, desserts and unsweetened breakfast cereals

● **Avoid syrups:** Eat canned fruit which is steeped in natural juice, not sugar syrup

● **Choose reduced-sugar products:** Read the labels on packaged foods to check the sugar content

BELIEVE IT OR NOT!

Here are some recipes for the same dish – but with fewer calories! Compare the recipes, the ingredients, the cooking methods *and* the final calorie counts.

CHOCOLATE MOUSSE LOW-CALORIE VERSION

1½ tablespoons cocoa
1 tablespoon cornflour
¾ pint/450ml skimmed milk
few drops of vanilla essence
artificial sweetener to taste
3 tablespoons hot water
¼ teaspoon coffee powder
1 sachet powdered gelatine
2 large egg whites
pinch of cream of tartar
4 teaspoons low-fat fromage frais
½ oz/15g milk chocolate, grated

1   Blend the cocoa and cornflour together with the milk. Add the vanilla essence and pour the cocoa mixture into a saucepan.
2   Bring to the boil, stirring all the time. Boil for 1-2 minutes and sweeten to taste.
3   Pour the hot water into a cup, add the coffee powder and gradually sprinkle in the gelatine.
4   Place the cup in a saucepan of simmering water until the gelatine dissolves.
5   Stir it into the chocolate sauce and set aside until cool and beginning to set.
6   Whisk the egg whites with the cream of tartar until they form soft peaks. Fold them into the setting mixture.
7   Spoon into 4 glasses and chill until set. Before serving, top with low-fat fromage frais and grated chocolate.

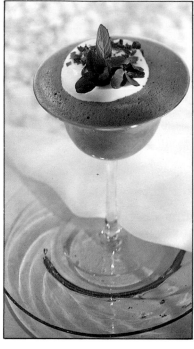

Preparation: 10 minutes

Cooking: 5 minutes plus chilling time

Serves 4   *90 calories per serving*

Selections per serving: ¼ Milk, 55 Optional Calories

CHOCOLATE MOUSSE HIGH-CALORIE VERSION

8oz/240g good-quality plain chocolate
1 tablespoon rum or orange liqueur
4 eggs, separated
2fl oz/60ml whipped cream

1   Break the chocolate into pieces and place in a basin over a small pan of gently simmering water until melted, stirring occasionally.
2   Remove the basin from the heat and beat in the rum and the egg yolks.

3   Beat the egg whites until they form soft peaks and gently fold into the chocolate mixture.
4   Spoon into 4 glasses and chill until firm. Before serving decorate with whipped cream.

Preparation: 10 minutes plus chilling time

Cooking: 5 minutes plus chilling time

Serves 4   *415 calories per serving*

Selections per serving:
1 Protein, 360 Optional Calories

LIGHT LASAGNE LOW-CALORIE VERSION

15oz/450g lean minced beef
1 teaspoon oil
1 medium onion, chopped
1 garlic clove, crushed
4oz/120g mushrooms, sliced
8oz/240g canned chopped tomatoes
¼ pint/150ml beef or vegetable stock
½ teaspoon dried oregano
salt and pepper
2 teaspoons cornflour
4oz/120g (6 sheets) precooked lasagne
1oz/30g mature Cheddar cheese, grated

For the cheese sauce:
1 tablespoon margarine
1oz/30g plain flour
½ pint/300ml skimmed milk
1oz/30g Cheddar cheese, grated

1   Shape the minced beef into small patties and place on the rack of a grill pan. Grill them, turning once, until the fat stops dripping.
2   Heat the oil and sauté the onion and garlic for 3 minutes, until softened. Add the beef, mushrooms, tomatoes and stock. Bring to the boil and simmer for 15-20 minutes. Add the oregano and season to taste.
3   Blend the cornflour with a

little water and stir into the mixture. Cook for 1-2 minutes until thickened, stirring. Remove from the heat.

4 Make the cheese sauce: place the margarine, flour and milk in a saucepan. Heat gently, stirring continuously with a wire whisk until the mixture boils and thickens. Add the cheese and season to taste.

5 Layer the minced beef mixture with the sheets of lasagne and cheese sauce, finishing with a layer of cheese sauce. Sprinkle with grated cheese and bake in a preheated oven at 190°C/375°F/Gas Mark 5 for 45 minutes, or until golden brown.

Preparation: 25 minutes

Cooking: 1 hour

Serves 4 *405 calories per serving*

Selections per serving:
1 Carbohydrate (Bread), 1 Fat, ¼ Milk, 3 Protein, 1½ Vegetable, 55 Optional Calories

LASAGNE
HIGH-CALORIE VERSION

1 medium onion, chopped
1 garlic clove, crushed
4 x ½ oz/15g slices streaky bacon, chopped
1 carrot, diced
1 celery stick, diced
2 tablespoons oil
1lb/480g minced beef
¼ pint/150ml red wine
salt and pepper
4fl oz/120ml milk
good pinch of ground nutmeg
1lb/480g tomatoes, skinned and chopped
1 tablespoon sugar
½ teaspoon dried oregano
4oz/120g (6 sheets) precooked lasagne
2oz/60g grated Parmesan cheese

For the cheese sauce:
1oz/30g butter or margarine
1oz/30g flour
½ pint/300ml milk
2oz/60g Cheddar cheese, grated

1 Sauté the onion, garlic, bacon, carrot and celery in the oil until tender. Add the minced beef and cook quickly until browned.

2 Add the wine and seasoning and cook over medium heat until most of the wine evaporates.

3 Add the milk and nutmeg and cook until reduced.

4 Add the tomatoes, sugar and oregano and bring to the boil. Reduce the heat to a bare simmer and cook very gently for about 2 hours, until the sauce is reduced and richly coloured.

5 Make the cheese sauce: melt the butter and stir in the flour. Cook for 2-3 minutes, and then gradually beat in the milk until the sauce is thick and glossy. Bring to the boil and then add the cheese and season to taste.

6 Layer the meat sauce, lasagne sheets and cheese sauce in an ovenproof dish, finishing with a layer of cheese sauce. Sprinkle with Parmesan cheese and bake in a preheated oven at 190°C/375°F/Gas Mark 5 for about 30 minutes, until golden.

Preparation: 25 minutes

Cooking: 2½ hours

Serves 4 *620 calories per serving*

Selections per serving:
1 Carbohydrate (Bread), 1½ Fat, ¼ Milk, 4 Protein, 1½ Vegetable, 190 Optional Calories

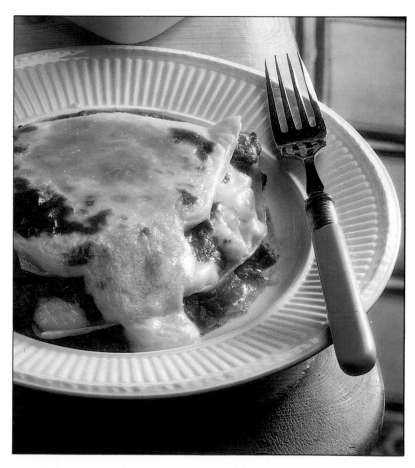

LIGHT LUNCHES AND SNACKS

SPICED PEANUT AND MUSHROOM SOUP

3oz/90g desiccated coconut
¾ pint/450ml boiling water
3 tablespoons chopped spring onions
½ pint/300ml vegetable stock
2 tablespoons lemon juice
1 teaspoon soft brown sugar
2oz/60g long-grain rice
2 tablespoons crunchy peanut butter
1 red pepper, deseeded and chopped
4oz/120g button mushrooms
½ teaspoon turmeric
½ teaspoon chilli powder

1   Place the coconut in a bowl, pour over the boiling water and leave to infuse for 20 minutes. Strain and reserve the liquid.

2   Place the spring onions, stock, coconut liquid, lemon juice, sugar, rice, peanut butter and red pepper in a large pan. Bring to the boil, then cover and simmer for 10 minutes.

3   Toss the mushrooms in the spices and add to the pan. Simmer for 5 minutes, or until rice is tender. Season to taste.

Preparation: 20 minutes plus infusing time

Cooking: 20 minutes

Serves 4   *100 calories per serving*

Selections per serving:
½ Carbohydrate (Bread), ½ Fat,
½ Protein, ½ Vegetable,
25 Optional Calories

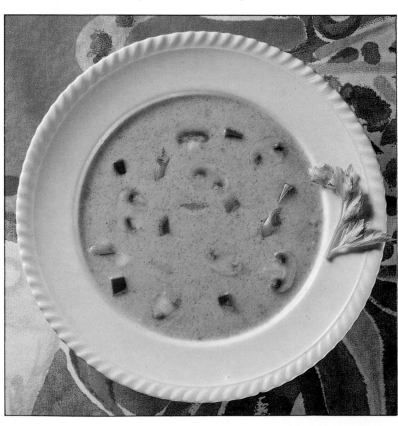

LEAN-LINE HERBY BURGERS

1lb/480g extra lean minced beef
2 tablespoons soy sauce
1 small onion, finely chopped
1 teaspoon dried mixed herbs
salt and pepper
2 teaspoons low-fat spread
2 teaspoons coarse-grain mustard
1 teaspoon horseradish relish
2 teaspoons vegetable oil
2 x 2oz/60g baps, split
salad leaves, tomatoes, and radishes
2 tablespoons chopped onion to garnish
8 teaspoons tomato ketchup

1   Mix together the beef, soy sauce, onion, herbs and seasoning. Divide the mixture into 4 portions and shape into burgers. Make a small hollow in the centre of each one.
2   Blend the low-fat spread with the mustard and horseradish and set aside.
3   Preheat the grill. Brush each burger with a little oil and grill for about 5 minutes on each side.
4   Place a burger on each of the halved baps on top of some salad leaves and sliced tomato. Spoon the mustard spread over the top and sprinkle with chopped onion. Serve with the remaining salad and tomato ketchup.

Preparation: 15 minutes

Cooking: 10 minutes

Serves 4   *350 calories per serving*

Selections per serving:
1 Carbohydrate (Bread), ½ Fat,
3 Protein, 1 Vegetable,
20 Optional Calories

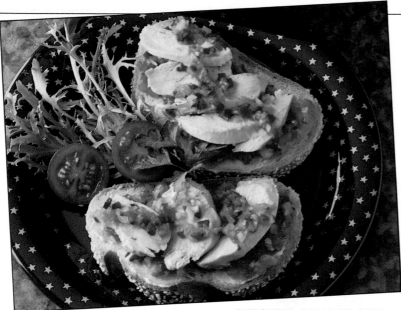

MEXICAN CHICKEN OPEN SANDWICH

1 shallot, finely chopped
2 tomatoes, chopped
½ small red pepper, deseeded and chopped
½ small fresh green chilli, deseeded and finely chopped
2 tablespoons tomato juice
2 x 1oz/30g slices bread
2 teaspoons low-fat spread
2oz/60g cooked chicken, sliced
salt and pepper
lettuce leaves to garnish

1 Mix together the shallot, tomatoes, red pepper, chilli and tomato juice to make a *salsa*.
2 Spread the slices of bread with the low-fat spread and arrange the sliced chicken on top. Place a tablespoon of salsa mixture on each open sandwich and sprinkle with salt and pepper.
3 Serve garnished with lettuce leaves, with the remaining salsa.

Preparation: 15 minutes

Serves 2 *130 calories per serving*

Selections per serving:
1 Carbohydrate (Bread), ½ Fat, 1 Protein, 1 Vegetable

CHICKEN, PRAWN AND PEPPER STIR-FRY

1 bunch spring onions, finely sliced
1 inch/2.5cm piece fresh root ginger, peeled and finely chopped
1 red pepper, 1 green pepper, 1 yellow pepper, deseeded and sliced
1 medium carrot, cut into match-stick strips
8oz/240g skinned, boned chicken breast, cut into strips
4 teaspoons sesame or vegetable oil
2oz/60g prawns
2 teaspoons light soy sauce
salt and pepper
1 tablespoon chopped coriander

1 Stir-fry the spring onions, ginger, peppers, carrot and chicken in the oil over high heat for 3-4 minutes until the chicken is cooked.
2 Stir in the prawns and soy sauce and season to taste. Cook for a further 30 seconds. Serve sprinkled with fresh coriander.

Preparation: 10 minutes

Cooking: 5 minutes

Serves 4 *145 calories per serving*

Selections per serving: 1 Fat, 1½ Protein, 1 Vegetable, 15 Optional Calories

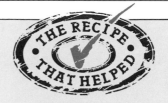

CHICKEN PASTA

As used by Debbie Jane Green, a successful Weight Watchers slimmer

1 medium onion, chopped
1 stick celery, chopped
3oz/90g mushrooms, chopped
1 garlic clove, crushed
1 tablespoon vegetable oil
8oz/240g canned tomatoes
½ teaspoon dried mixed herbs
salt and pepper
2oz/60g cooked chicken, cut into strips
3oz/90g cooked pasta shapes
1oz/30g Cheddar cheese, grated

1 Sauté the onion, celery, mushrooms and garlic in the oil for 5 minutes.
2 Stir in the tomatoes, herbs and seasoning and cook gently for 5 minutes.
3 Add the chicken and pasta. Stir well and transfer to an ovenproof dish.
4 Sprinkle with grated cheese and place under a hot grill until golden brown.

Preparation: 15 minutes

Cooking: 15 minutes

Serves 2 *255 calories per serving*

Selections per serving:
½ Carbohydrate (Bread), 1½ Fat, 1½ Protein, 2 Vegetable

LIGHT LUNCHES AND SNACKS

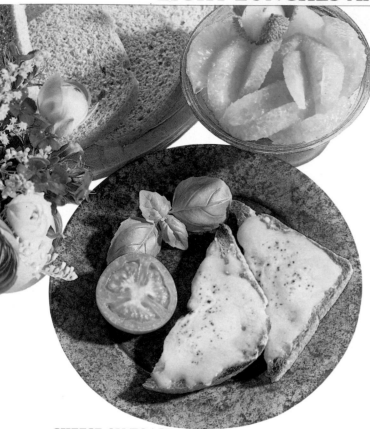

Add the chicken and the rice mixture, mixing well. Season to taste with salt and pepper, and garnish with lemon and parsley.

Preparation: 10 minutes

Serves 2 *380 calories per serving*

Selections per serving:
1 Carbohydrate (Bread), 1 Fat, 2 Fruit, 2 Protein, 20 Optional Calories

STUFFED JACKET POTATOES

1 x 8oz/240g potato
1½ oz/45g cooked ham, chopped
1 tablespoon chopped spring onion
½ oz/15g mature Cheddar cheese, grated
2 tablespoons skimmed milk
salt and pepper

1 Pierce the potato skin 2 or 3 times and bake in a hot oven at 200°C/400°F/Gas Mark 6 for 45 minutes, or until cooked.
2 Cut the potato in half and scoop out the middle. Mash well and mix in the ham, spring onion, cheese and milk. Season to taste.
3 Pile back into the potato skins and place on a baking sheet. Pop back into the oven for 5-10 minutes until golden.

Preparation: 5 minutes

Cooking: 55 minutes

Serves 1 285 *calories*

Selections:
2 Carbohydrate (Bread),
2 Protein, 10 Optional Calories

Alternative Filling
1 tablespoon low-fat soft cheese
2 teaspoons chopped chives
2oz/60g peeled prawns
salt and pepper

1 Mash the soft cheese and

CHEESE ON TOAST

1 slice reduced-calorie bread
1 teaspoon French mustard
1oz/30g mature Cheddar cheese, sliced
½ tomato
fresh basil to garnish

1 Toast the bread lightly and spread with the mustard.
2 Cover with the cheese and grill until bubbling. Serve with tomato, garnished with basil.

Preparation and cooking:
5 minutes

Serves 1 *160 calories*

Selections:
½ Carbohydrate (Bread),
1 Protein, ½ Vegetable

CARIBBEAN CHICKEN SALAD

6oz/180g cooked long-grain rice
2oz/60g canned pineapple, drained and chopped
1 medium banana, sliced
3oz/90g seedless grapes, halved
4 teaspoons lemon juice
½oz/15g sultanas
4 teaspoons desiccated coconut
2 tablespoons low-fat natural yogurt
4 teaspoons low-calorie mayonnaise
4oz/120g cooked chicken, roughly chopped
salt and pepper
lemon slices and parsley to garnish

1 Mix together the rice, fresh fruit and lemon juice.
2 Combine the sultanas, coconut, yogurt and mayonnaise.

chives with the cooked potato. Mix in the prawns. Season and pile back into the potato skins.
2 Pop back into the oven for 5 minutes to heat through.

Serves 1 *245 calories*

Selections:
2 Carbohydrate (Bread),
1 Protein, 15 Optional Calories

CHICKEN AND SWEETCORN SOUP

2 teaspoons margarine
1 small onion, finely chopped
½ small red pepper, finely chopped
3oz/90g skinned and boned chicken breast, chopped
¾ pint/450ml chicken stock
3oz/90g canned sweetcorn kernels
½ teaspoon finely grated lemon rind
2 teaspoons cornflour
salt and pepper
fine strips of lemon rind and fresh herbs to garnish

1 Melt the margarine in a saucepan and sauté the onion and pepper over gentle heat for about 5 minutes, until the onion is soft and translucent.
2 Add the chicken and cook, stirring, for 2-3 minutes.
3 Pour in the chicken stock and bring to the boil. Cover the pan and simmer for 10 minutes.

4 Add the sweetcorn and lemon rind, and cook for 5 minutes.
5 Blend the cornflour with a little cold water and mix into the soup, stirring until it thickens. Cook gently for 1 minute.
6 Check the seasoning and serve garnished with lemon rind and herbs.

Preparation: 5 minutes

Cooking: 30 minutes

Serves 2 *160 calories per serving*

Selections per serving:
½ Carbohydrate (Bread), 1 Fat,
1 Protein, ½ Vegetable,
15 Optional Calories

PRAWN PITTA PARCEL

1 mini wholemeal pitta
2 teaspoons low-calorie mayonnaise
1 teaspoon lemon juice
1oz/30g beansprouts
1 teaspoon chopped chives
2oz/60g peeled prawns
salt and pepper
shredded lettuce

1 Place the pitta under a hot grill for about 2 minutes, turning once until lightly crisp.
2 Blend the mayonnaise and lemon juice, and stir in the beansprouts, chives and prawns. Season to taste.
3 Slit along one side of the

pitta. Fill with shredded lettuce and the prawn mayonnaise mixture.

Preparation: 5 minutes

Serves 1 *160 calories per serving*

Selections: 1 Carbohydrate (Bread), 1 Fat, 1 Protein, ½ Vegetable,

HOT CHEESE AND GARLIC BREAD

As used by Linda Dawson, a successful Weight Watchers slimmer

1 x 6oz/180g French bread stick, cut into 12 thin slices
2 tablespoons low-fat spread
2 garlic cloves, crushed
2 tablespoons chopped fresh parsley
3oz/90g mature Cheddar cheese, grated

1 Preheat the oven to 200°C/400°F/Gas Mark 6.
2 Place the slices of bread on a baking sheet. Mix the low-fat spread with the garlic and parsley, and spread a little over each slice.
3 Sprinkle with the cheese and bake in oven for 6-8 minutes until bubbling and golden.

Preparation: 5 minutes

Cooking: 6-8 minutes

Serves 6 (2 each) *165 calories per serving*

Selections per serving:
1 Carbohydrate (Bread), ½ Fat, ½ Protein

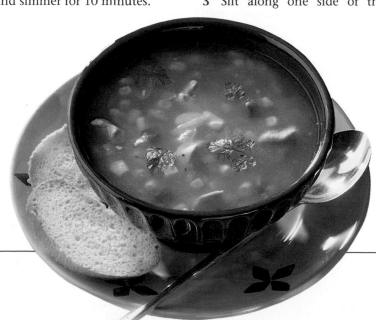

MAIN MEALS WITH FISH

THAI GRILLED FISH

1 x 12oz/360g fish, e.g. snapper or
trout, scaled and gutted
2 tablespoons vegetable oil
1 tablespoon soy sauce
1 tablespoon lime or lemon juice
1 tablespoon cornflour
½ pint/300ml cold water
2 spring onions, cut in diagonal
chunks
1 garlic clove, peeled and finely
chopped
1 inch/2.5cm piece of root ginger,
sliced thinly
1 small red pepper, deseeded and
sliced
1 green pepper, deseeded and sliced
4oz/120g oyster or large button
mushrooms, sliced
1 tablespoon ground turmeric
salt and pepper
fresh coriander or parsley to garnish

1 Wash the fish well under
running cold water. Pat dry with
kitchen paper and brush with a
little of the oil. Place on the rack
of a grill pan, and preheat the grill.
2 Blend the soy sauce with the
lime juice and cornflour and
gradually add the cold water, stirring well until smooth.
3 Grill the fish for about 5
minutes on each side, turning
carefully. Place the cooked fish
on a serving plate. Keep warm.
4 Heat the remaining oil in a
wok or frying pan and stir-fry the
onions, garlic, ginger, peppers
and mushrooms for about 3
minutes, until tender but still
crisp.
5 Stir in the turmeric and cook
for 1 more minute. Add the soy
sauce mixture, stirring well until
thickened, and season to taste.
Spoon over the grilled fish and
serve garnished with fresh herbs.

Preparation: 15 minutes

Cooking: 15 minutes

Serves 2 *290 calories per serving*

Selections per serving: 2 Fat,
2 Protein, 1½ Vegetable,
55 Optional Calories

SALMON IN A PARCEL

2 x 4oz/120g salmon steaks
1 carrot, cut into matchstick strips
1 leek, cut into thin strips
few slices of fresh ginger
1 tablespoon soy sauce
½ garlic clove, crushed
½ teaspoon Worcestershire sauce
freshly ground black pepper
2 sprigs fresh parsley, chopped

1 Cut 2 pieces of greaseproof
paper or foil large enough to
enclose the salmon steaks. Place
the fish on top and cover with
the vegetables and ginger.
2 Mix together the soy sauce,
garlic and Worcestershire sauce.
Pour over the fish and grind
plenty of black pepper on top.
3 Fold the paper or foil over
and secure the edges to make 2
neat parcels and place on a
baking tray.
4 Bake in a preheated oven at
180°C/350°F/Gas Mark 4 for 15-
20 minutes.
5 Carefully unwrap the fish and
check that it is cooked. Transfer
to a warm serving dish and sprinkle with parsley.

Preparation: 10 minutes

Cooking: 15-20 minutes

Serves 2 *230 calories per serving*

Selections per serving:
3 Protein, ½ Vegetable,

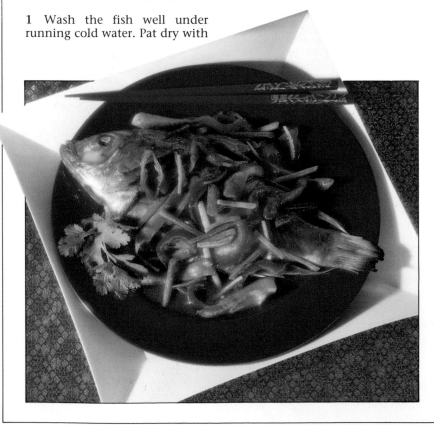

MEDITERRANEAN BAKED FISH

4 teaspoons vegetable oil
1 small onion, chopped
2 medium courgettes, sliced
1 red pepper, deseeded and sliced
8oz/240g canned chopped tomatoes
4 teaspoons tomato purée
¼ pint/150ml vegetable stock
4 x 5oz/150g cod cutlets
1 teaspoon dried oregano
salt and pepper

1 Heat the oil and stir-fry the onion, courgettes and pepper for 3-4 minutes. Add the tomatoes.
2 Mix the tomato purée with the stock and add to the vegetables. Simmer for 2 minutes; transfer to an ovenproof dish.
3 Lay the fish cutlets on top and sprinkle with oregano. Season, cover and bake in a preheated oven at 190°C/375°F/Gas Mark 5 for 20 minutes.

Preparation: 15 minutes

Cooking: 30 minutes

Serves 4 *175 calories per serving*

Selections per serving: 1 Fat, 3 Protein, 1½ Vegetable

MIXED FISH CASSEROLE

10oz/300g mixed white fish, e.g. boned monkfish, skinned haddock and cod fillet
2 teaspoons vegetable oil
1 garlic clove, crushed
1 medium onion, chopped
8oz/240g canned chopped tomatoes
4fl oz/120ml dry white wine
good pinch of dried thyme
1 tablespoon chopped fresh parsley
salt and pepper
4oz/120g peeled prawns

1 Cut the monkfish (if using) into cubes. Cut the haddock and cod fillets into strips.
2 Heat the oil in a flameproof casserole and stir-fry the garlic and onion for 3-4 minutes.

TUNA AND PASTA MIX

As used by Penny Smith, a successful Weight Watchers slimmer

3oz/90g pasta spirals
salt
1 medium orange, segmented
2 inch/5cm wedge of cucumber, diced
1 stick of celery, diced
½ red pepper, deseeded and diced
6oz/180g drained canned tuna, flaked
2 ½fl oz/75ml low-fat natural yogurt
1 tablespoon orange juice
2 teaspoons lemon juice
½ teaspoon Dijon mustard
1 tablespoon chopped parsley

1 Cook the pasta in boiling salted water until tender (*al dente*). Then drain well.
2 Mix the orange with the cucumber, celery, pepper and tuna and stir in the pasta.
3 Blend the yogurt with the orange and lemon juice and mustard. Pour over the pasta, and toss gently with parsley.

Preparation: 15 minutes

Cooking: 10-15 minutes

Serves 2 300 *calories per serving*

Selections per serving:
1½ Carbohydrate (Bread),
½ Fruit, ¼ Milk, 1½ Protein,
1 Vegetable

3 Add the tomatoes, wine and herbs. Bring to the boil, add the prepared fish and seasoning.
4 Cover and bake in a preheated oven at 180°C/350°F/Gas Mark 4 for 20 minutes.
5 Add the prawns, cover and return to the oven for a further 10 minutes.

Preparation: 10 minutes

Cooking: 40 minutes

Serves 4 *145 calories per serving*

Selections per serving: ½ Fat, 1½ Protein, 1 Vegetable, 25 Optional Calories

THE RECIPE THAT HELPED

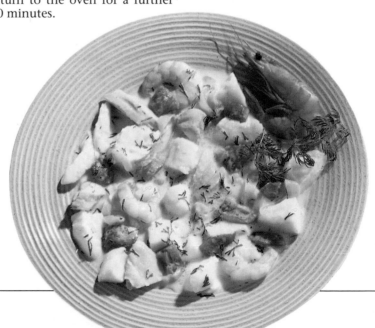

MAIN MEALS WITH MEAT AND POULTRY

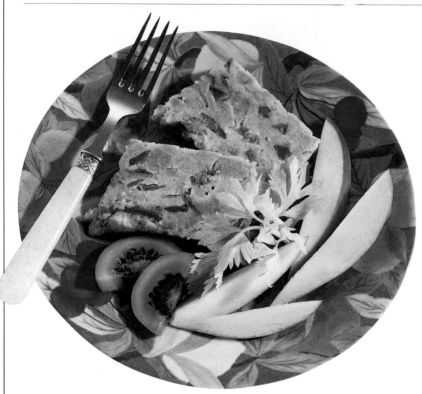

SPICY MARINATED LAMB KEBABS

5fl oz/150ml low-fat natural yogurt
1 teaspoon ground cumin
2 teaspoons ground turmeric
finely grated zest of ½ lime
1 garlic clove, crushed
2 teaspoons sesame oil
salt and pepper
1lb/480g boned lean leg of lamb

1 Mix the yogurt, ground cumin and turmeric, grated lime zest, garlic and sesame oil together in a bowl, and season with salt and pepper.
2 Cut the lamb into cubes and stir into the yogurt marinade, making sure that it is well coated. Leave to marinate in the refrigerator for at least 4-5 hours to absorb the flavour of the marinade.
3 Thread the lamb on to 4 kebab skewers and place them on the rack of a grill pan (or barbecue). Brush the lamb kebabs with the remaining marinade.
4 Place the kebabs under a hot grill, turning occasionally until thoroughly cooked. Serve them with a crisp green salad.

Preparation: 10 minutes plus marinating time
Cooking: 10 – 12 minutes
Serves 4 *220 calories per serving*
Selections per serving: ½ Fat, ¼ Milk, 3 Protein

CARIBBEAN DINNER

10oz/300g canned ham, chopped
4oz/120g green pepper, deseeded and chopped
2oz/60g onion, finely chopped
2oz/60g fresh breadcrumbs
salt and pepper
pinch of paprika
pinch of ground mace
4 teaspoons margarine, softened
2 eggs, beaten
4 x 1oz/30g pineapple rings in natural juice, drained and cut in half
1 passionfruit and 1 medium mango, sliced (optional)

1 Mix the ham with the pepper, onion and breadcrumbs. Add the seasoning, ground paprika and mace.
2 Add the margarine and eggs to bind the mixture.
3 Line a 2lb/1kg loaf tin with non-stick silicone paper. Arrange 4 of the pineapple halves in the base of the tin, and 2 halves up each side. Spoon in the meat mixture and smooth the top to make it level.
4 Bake in a preheated oven at 180°C/350°F/Gas Mark 4 for 1 hour. Turn the meat loaf out of the tin and serve cut into slices, hot or cold, decorated with mango slices and passionfruit.

Preparation: 10 minutes
Cooking: 1 hour
Serves 4 *380 calories per serving*
Selections per serving:
½ Carbohydrate (Bread), 1 Fat, ½ Fruit, 3 Protein, ½ Vegetable, 20 Optional Calories

PORK KEBABS

1lb/480g pork fillet or tenderloin
5fl oz/150ml low-fat natural yogurt
3 onion slices
finely grated zest of ¼ lemon
1½ teaspoons chopped sage
2 tablespoons oil
1 medium onion, cut into 8 wedges
½ small red pepper, deseeded and cut
into chunks
½ small yellow pepper, deseeded and
cut into chunks
4 small courgettes, cut in half

1 Cut the pork into 1-1½ inch/2.5-3.5cm cubes and place in a bowl. Mix the yogurt with the onion slices, lemon zest, sage and 2 teaspoons of the oil.
2 Pour the yogurt marinade over the pork and mix well. Cover and place in the refrigerator for several hours or overnight.
3 Remove the onion rings from the marinade and thread the pork on to 4 kebab skewers alternately with the onion wedges, peppers and courgettes.
4 Brush the pork with the rest of the marinade, and then brush

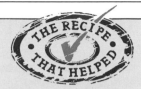

BLUE CHEESE BEEF

As used by Julia Westgarth, a successful Weight Watchers slimmer

1lb/480g minced lean beef
1 onion, chopped
2 teaspoons vegetable oil
4 teaspoons plain flour
8oz/240g canned chopped
tomatoes
½ teaspoon dried marjoram
2oz/60g mushrooms, sliced
2 tablespoons beef stock
salt and pepper
8oz/240g frozen leaf spinach
2 teaspoons cornflour
½ pint/300ml skimmed milk
2oz/60g blue cheese

1 Grill the minced beef until the fat stops dripping.
2 Stir-fry the onion in the oil for 5 minutes. Stir in the flour.
3 Add the tomatoes, marjoram, mushrooms, stock, beef and seasoning.
4 Bring to the boil, then simmer, covered for 10 minutes. Simmer uncovered for 10 more minutes.
5 Cook the spinach and drain well.
6 Blend the cornflour with a little milk. Heat the remaining milk and stir into the cornflour paste. Bring to the boil, stirring, and boil for 2 minutes. Add the cheese.
7 Spread the spinach over the base of an ovenproof dish and cover with the beef mixture. Top with the sauce and bake at 200°C/400°F/Gas Mark 6 for 20 minutes.

Preparation: 15 minutes

Cooking: 55 minutes

Serves 4 *325 calories per serving*

Selections per serving: ½ Fat, ¼ Milk, 3 Protein, 2 Vegetable, 45 Optional Calories

the vegetables with some of the remaining oil.
5 Cook the kebabs under a hot grill (or on the barbecue), turning occasionally and brushing with oil until cooked. Serve with a crisp green salad.

Preparation: 10 minutes plus marinating time

Cooking: 10-12 minutes

Serves 4 *295 calories per serving*

Selections per serving: 1½ Fat, ¼ Milk, 3 Protein, 1 Vegetable

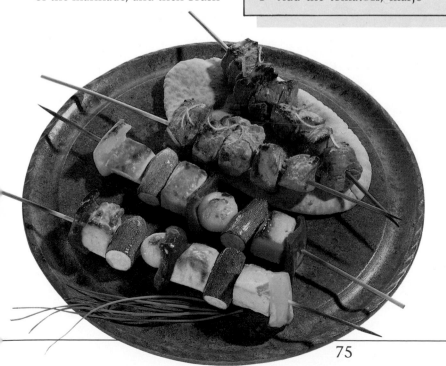

MAIN MEALS WITH MEAT AND POULTRY

SWEET AND SOUR CHICKEN

2 teaspoons oil
1 garlic clove, crushed
10oz/300g skinned and boned
chicken, sliced
1 medium onion, sliced
1 small carrot, cut into matchstick
pieces
3oz/90g mangetout, sliced in half
½ pint/300ml chicken stock
3 medium tomatoes, skinned and
quartered
1 tablespoon cornflour
1 tablespoon caster sugar
2 tablespoons vinegar
2 tablespoons light soy sauce
salt and pepper
12oz/360g cooked rice to serve

1　Heat the oil in a large saucepan and sauté the garlic for 2 minutes without browning. Add the chicken pieces and cook for 2-3 minutes, stirring continuously, until sealed on all sides.

2　Add the onion, carrot and mangetout, then pour in the chicken stock. Bring to the boil, reduce the heat and simmer gently for 20-30 minutes until the chicken is tender. Add the tomatoes and stir gently.
3　Blend the cornflour, sugar, vinegar and soy sauce. Stir into the chicken and vegetables and cook for 2-3 minutes until thickened. Season to taste.
4　Serve in bowls with the hot cooked rice.

Preparation: 15 minutes

Cooking: 40 minutes

Serves 4 *260 calories per serving*

Selections per serving:
1 Carbohydrate (Bread), ½ Fat,
2 Protein, 1½ Vegetable,
25 Optional Calories

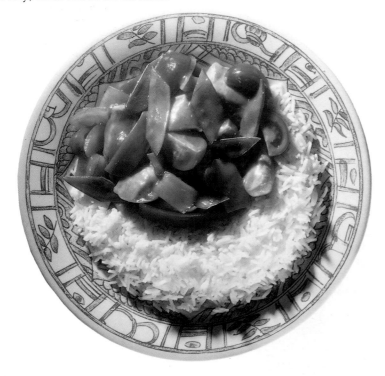

CHILLI CHICKEN STIR-FRY

1 tablespoon oil
12oz/360g skinned and boned
chicken breasts, cubed
3oz/90g peanuts
¼ cucumber, cubed
4oz/120g mangetout
1 garlic clove, crushed
1 teaspoon tomato purée
1 tablespoon soy sauce
2 teaspoons chilli sauce
3 tablespoons water

1　Heat the oil in a wok.
2　Add the chicken and stir-fry until lightly browned.
3　Add the peanuts, cucumber, mangetout and garlic and stir-fry for 1 minute.
4　Add the remaining ingredients and bring to the boil. Cover and cook for 5 minutes, until the chicken is tender.

Preparation: 10 minutes

Cooking: 10 minutes

Serves 4 *260 calories per serving*

Selections per serving: 2 Fat,
3 Protein, ½ Vegetable,
15 Optional Calories

CHOPS WITH GRILLED PEPPERS

1 red and 1 yellow pepper
1 medium onion, quartered and
separated into chunks
2 tablespoons chopped fresh parsley
1 teaspoon grated onion
grated rind of 1 small lemon
1oz/30g slice bread, crust removed
salt and pepper
4 x 5oz/150g lamb loin chops,
trimmed of fat

1　Grill the peppers with the onion chunks until they start to look charred. Peel and slice the peppers.
2　Mix the parsley, grated onion

and lemon rind together. Soak the bread quickly in cold water. Squeeze dry, crumble into the parsley mixture and season.
3 Press the stuffing into each chop and secure with wooden cocktail sticks.
4 Grill for 6-8 minutes each side. Serve with the vegetables.

Preparation: 15 minutes

Cooking: 6-8 minutes

Serves 4 *295 calories per serving*

Selections per serving:
3 Protein, ¾ Vegetable,
20 Optional Calories.

SLIM SHEPHERD'S PIE

15oz/450g lean minced lamb
1 large onion, chopped
2oz/60g mushrooms, sliced
2 carrots, diced
1 turnip, diced
1 tablespoon plain flour
½ pint/300ml vegetable stock
1 bay leaf
½ teaspoon mixed herbs
salt and pepper
1½ lb/720g cooked potatoes
2 teaspoons margarine

1 Grill the minced lamb until the fat stops dripping.
2 Crumble the lamb into a large saucepan to break it up. Add the onion and dry-fry for 3 minutes. Stir in the mushrooms, carrots and turnip.
3 Sprinkle the flour into the pan and cook, stirring, for 1 minute. Gradually blend in the stock and then bring to the boil so that the mixture thickens. Add the bay leaf, herbs and seasoning, and simmer for 25 minutes.
4 Mash the potatoes with the margarine and pepper.
5 Transfer the mince mixture to an ovenproof dish. Remove the bay leaf and pile the cooked potato on top. Place in a pre-heated oven at 200°C/400°F/Gas Mark 6 for 10-15 minutes.

Preparation: 20 minutes

Cooking: 1 hour

Serves 4 *370 calories per serving*

Selections per serving:
1½ Carbohydrate (Bread) ½ Fat,
3 Protein, 1½ Vegetable,
10 Optional Calories

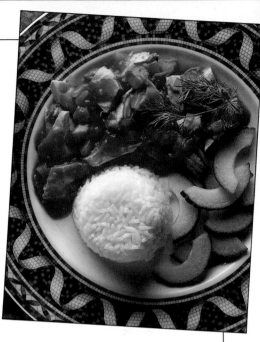

CHICKEN CURRY

1 medium onion, chopped
2 garlic cloves, chopped
2 teaspoons oil
2 teaspoons garam masala
½ teaspoon ground ginger
½ teaspoon chilli powder
14oz/420g canned tomatoes
½ pint/300ml chicken stock
1lb/480g cooked chicken, skinned and roughly chopped
salt and pepper
12oz/360g cooked rice to serve
sliced cucumber to garnish

1 Sauté the onion and garlic in the oil until soft and translucent.
2 Stir in the spices and cook, stirring, for 1 minute.
3 Add the tomatoes and stock, cover and simmer for 20 minutes.
4 Add the chicken and simmer, uncovered, for a few minutes.
5 Season and serve with rice and cucumber.

Preparation: 10 minutes

Cooking: 30 minutes

Serves 4 *310 calories per serving*

Selections per serving:
1 Carbohydrate (Bread), ½ Fat,
3 Protein, 2 Vegetable,
65 Optional Calories

CUMIN CHICKEN

As used by Sue Callaway, a successful Weight Watchers slimmer

4 teaspoons vegetable oil
1½ teaspoons cumin seeds
2 teaspoons finely chopped fresh root ginger
8oz/240g canned water chestnuts, drained and sliced
1 red pepper, deseeded and cut into strips
8 spring onions, cut into ½ inch/1.25 cm pieces
6oz/180g canned sweetcorn
14oz/420g chicken breast fillets, cut into ½ inch/1.25cm strips
2 teaspoons flour
6fl oz/180ml chicken stock

1 Heat the oil and stir-fry the cumin seeds until they pop.
2 Add the ginger, vegetables and chicken. Stir-fry for 2-3 minutes.
3 Stir in the flour and add the stock. Bring to the boil, stirring. Cover and simmer for 10 minutes.

Preparation: 10 minutes

Cooking: 20 minutes

Serves 4 *230 calories per serving*

Selections per serving:
1 Carbohydrate (Bread), 1 Fat,
3 Protein, ½ Vegetable,
10 Optional Calories

VEGETARIAN MAIN MEALS

VEGETABLE RISOTTO

1 tablespoon oil (preferably olive oil)
1 medium onion, chopped
1 red pepper, deseeded and chopped
1 medium carrot, diced
2 garlic cloves, crushed
8oz/240g risotto rice, e.g. arborio
1¾ pints/1 litre hot vegetable stock
3 tablespoons dry white wine or vermouth
3oz/90g baby sweetcorn
2oz/60g button mushrooms, sliced
8 thin asparagus spears
salt and ground black pepper
1oz/30g grated Parmesan cheese

1   Heat the oil in a large frying pan and sauté the onion, pepper, carrot and garlic until soft.
2   Add the rice and cook gently for 2 minutes until opaque.
3   Stir in about one-quarter of the vegetable stock and the wine. Add the sweetcorn, mushrooms and asparagus and cook gently

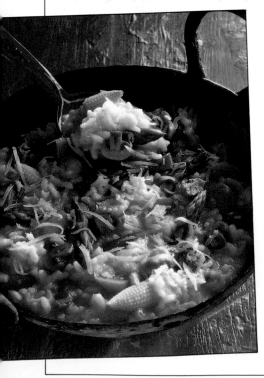

until the liquid is absorbed.
4   Add some more stock, stirring occasionally. Keep adding the stock until it has all been absorbed and the risotto is creamy.
5   Season to taste with salt and freshly ground black pepper and sprinkle with grated Parmesan.

Preparation: 10 minutes
Cooking: 30-35 minutes
Serves 4   *270 calories per serving*
Selections per serving:
2 Carbohydrate (Bread), ½ Fat, 1 Vegetable, 55 Optional Calories

RATATOUILLE

12oz/360g aubergine, cubed
salt
2 tablespoons vegetable or olive oil
1 clove garlic, finely chopped
1 medium onion, chopped
1 medium red pepper, deseeded and sliced
1 medium green pepper, deseeded and sliced
12oz/360g courgettes, thickly sliced
14oz/420g canned chopped tomatoes
1 tablespoon tomato purée
½ teaspoon dried basil or 2 teaspoons chopped fresh basil
2 teaspoons chopped parsley or sprig of basil to garnish (optional)

1   Sprinkle the aubergine with salt and leave to drain for 20-30 minutes to exude its bitter juices. Rinse well and pat dry.
2   Heat the oil in a flameproof casserole. Add the garlic, onion and peppers and sauté for 2-3 minutes.
3   Mix in the aubergines, courgettes, tomatoes, tomato purée and basil.
4   Cover the casserole and place in a preheated oven at 180°C/

350°F/Gas Mark 4 for 45 minutes. Serve sprinkled with parsley or garnished with basil.

Preparation: 20-30 minutes
Cooking: 50 minutes
Serves 4   *110 calories per serving*
Selections per serving: 1½ Fat, 4 Vegetable

MACARONI CHEESE AND CAULIFLOWER

10oz/300g cooked cauliflower florets
6oz/180g cooked macaroni
4oz/120g button mushrooms, sliced
salt and pepper to taste
paprika to garnish
For the cheese sauce:
2 tablespoons margarine
2 tablespoons plain flour
½ pint/300ml skimmed milk
4oz/120g Cheddar cheese, grated
dash of Worcestershire sauce or pinch of nutmeg

1   To make the sauce: melt the margarine in a saucepan. Blend in the flour, and then the milk. Cook, stirring, until thickened. Stir in the cheese and Worcestershire sauce or nutmeg.
2   Mix together the cauliflower, macaroni, mushrooms, salt and pepper with the cheese sauce. Put in a 2-pint/1.2 litre ovenproof dish and sprinkle with paprika.
3   Cover the dish and bake at 180°C/350°F/Gas Mark 4 for 30 minutes. Uncover and bake for 5 minutes until brown.

Preparation: 10 minutes
Cooking: 45 minutes
Serves 2   *530 calories per serving*
Selections per serving:
1 Carbohydrate (Bread), 2 Fat, ½ Milk, 2 Protein, 2 Vegetable, 70 Optional Calories

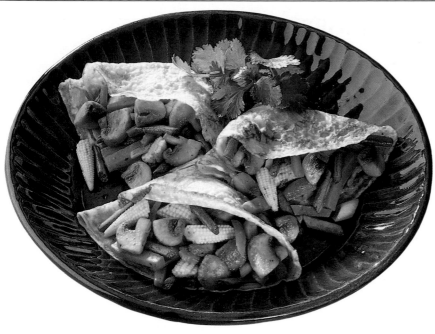

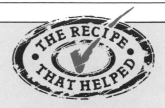

TWO CHEESE PASTA

As used by Lynda Jones, a successful Weight Watchers slimmer

6oz/180g pasta shapes
salt
1½ tablespoons margarine
4 spring onions, cut into thick diagonal slices
1 red pepper, deseeded and cut into strips
1 green pepper, deseeded and cut into strips
12oz/360g low-fat soft cheese
4oz/120g Gorgonzola cheese, crumbled
4 tomatoes, sliced
1 tablespoon chopped parsley

1 Cook the pasta in boiling salted water for about 12 minutes. Drain well.
2 Meanwhile, heat the margarine and stir-fry the vegetables for 5 minutes. Reduce the heat and stir in the two cheeses. Cook for 1 minute, stirring.
3 Stir the drained hot pasta into the cheese sauce and pile on to a warm plate. Serve with the sliced tomatoes, sprinkled with parsley.

Preparation: 5 minutes

Cooking: 12 minutes

Serves 4 *380 calories per serving*

Selections per serving:
1½ Bread, 2½ Protein, 1 Fat, 1½ Vegetable, 5 Optional Calories

SESAME PANCAKES WITH STIR-FRIED VEGETABLES

4oz/120g plain flour
pinch of salt
1 egg
½ pint/300ml skimmed milk
2 teaspoons oil
4 teaspoons sesame seeds
For the filling:
2 teaspoons oil
1 large carrot, cut into matchstick strips
4oz/120g dwarf green beans, sliced
1 bunch spring onions, sliced
3oz/90g baby sweetcorn
4oz/120g mushrooms, sliced
½ teaspoon five spice powder (optional)
salt and pepper

1 To make the pancakes: sift the flour and salt into a large bowl. Add the egg and milk and beat well to make a smooth batter.
2 Heat a small heavy-based frying pan and add a few drops of oil for each pancake.
3 Pour a little batter into the hot pan, tilting the pan to spread the mixture evenly over the base. Sprinkle ½ teaspoon of sesame seeds over the surface before the mixture sets, and then carefully flip the pancake over to cook the other side.
4 Make all 8 pancakes in this way and keep them warm, covered with foil, while you prepare the stir-fried vegetable filling.
5 To make the filling: heat the oil in a large frying pan or wok. Add the carrot, beans, spring onions and sweetcorn, and stir-fry for 2 minutes.
6 Add the mushrooms and five spice powder and stir-fry for 1-2 minutes. Season to taste with salt and pepper and divide the stir-fried vegetables between the warm pancakes. Fold over and serve immediately.

Preparation: 20 minutes

Cooking: 20 minutes

Serves 4 *230 calories per serving*

Selections per serving:
1 Carbohydrate (Bread), 1 Fat, ¼ Milk, 1 Vegetable, 50 Optional Calories

DESSERTS

EXOTIC FRUIT PAVLOVA

2 large egg whites
pinch of cream of tartar
4oz/120g caster sugar
1oz/30g ground almonds
4oz/120g curd cheese
6oz/180g fromage frais (8% fat)
1lb/480g mixed fresh berries

1 Whisk the egg whites together with the cream of tartar until peaking. Gradually add about half the sugar, one tablespoon at a time, whisking well after each addition until the mixture peaks.

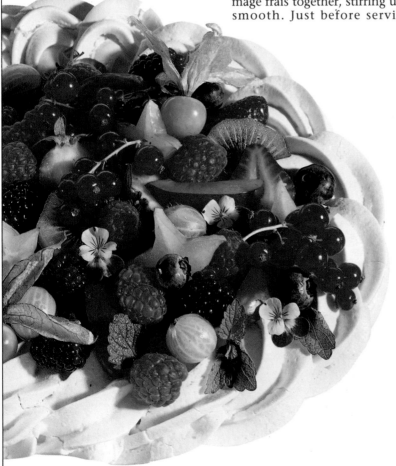

2 Mix the remaining sugar with the ground nuts and carefully fold into the whisked mixture.
3 Lay a piece of non-stick baking parchment on a baking sheet and spoon the meringue mixture on to it. Carefully spread the meringue into an 8 inch/20cm circle and then make a slight dip in the centre. With a fork swirl the edge into several peaks.
4 Cook at 140°C/275°F/Gas Mark 1 for 1 hour. Turn the oven off and leave for several hours until completely cold.
5 Mix the curd cheese and fromage frais together, stirring until smooth. Just before serving, spread this mixture over the meringue and top with the berries.

Preparation: 15 minutes
Cooking: 1 hour plus cooling
Serves 8 *165 calories per serving*
Selections per serving: ½ Fruit, ½ Protein, 90 Optional Calories

CHOCOLATE APRICOT CHEESECAKE

3oz/90g margarine
1½oz/45g chocolate
2 teaspoons cocoa
12 large digestive biscuits
10oz/300g curd cheese
6oz/180g low-fat fromage frais
8oz/240g drained canned apricots,
6 tablespoons natural juice reserved
2 tablespoons frozen concentrated
orange juice, thawed
1½ tablespoons sugar
1 sachet powdered gelatine
2 egg whites
pinch of cream of tartar

1 Melt the margarine in a small saucepan. Break half the chocolate into a cup and stand in a saucepan of simmering water until melted.
2 Stir the cocoa into the melted margarine, add the melted chocolate and mix well.
3 Break the remaining chocolate into the cup and set aside.
4 Crush the biscuits into crumbs and stir into the margarine and chocolate mixture.
5 Spoon the crumb mixture into an 8 inch/20cm springform tin and spread firmly over the base.
6 Place the curd cheese, fromage frais, apricots and half of the reserved juice, orange juice and sugar in a food processor or blender, and process to a purée
7 Pour the remaining juice into

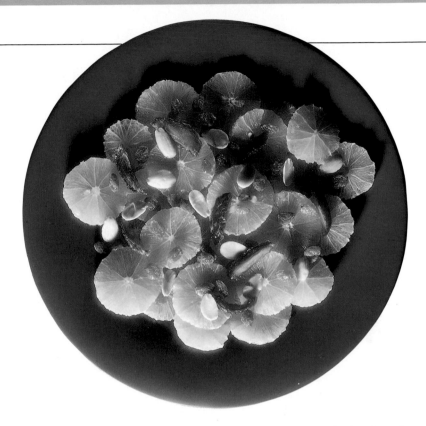

a cup and sprinkle in the gelatine. Stir well and then place in a saucepan of simmering water until the gelatine has dissolved.

8 Add the dissolved gelatine to the purée and process once again. Pour into a bowl and chill until thick and beginning to set.

9 Whisk the egg whites and cream of tartar until they form soft peaks, and gently fold into the purée. Pour into the tin over the biscuit base and smooth the surface.

10 Stand the cup of chocolate in a pan of simmering water until melted. Using a fork, drizzle the melted chocolate over the top of the cheesecake and swirl attractively.

11 Chill well until completely set. Remove from the tin to serve.

Preparation: 25 minutes plus setting and chilling time

Serves 12 *200 calories per serving*

Selections per serving:
1 Carbohydrate (Bread), 1½ Fat, 85 Optional Calories

MOROCCAN ORANGE PLATTER

4 medium oranges
1 tablespoon soft brown sugar
2 inch/5cm piece of cinnamon stick
2oz/60g fresh or dried dates, pitted
1oz/30g sultanas
½ oz/15g blanched almonds, cut into slivers

1 Pare the rind from 2 oranges, using a potato peeler or sharp knife. Place in a saucepan with the sugar, cinnamon stick and ¼ pint/150ml water. Heat and simmer gently for 10-15 minutes to reduce. Cool and discard the rind and cinnamon.

2 Use a serrated knife to remove all the peel and pith from the oranges. Slice them crossways and arrange on a large platter.

3 Slice the dates into thin slivers and scatter them over the oranges with the sultanas and almonds.

4 Pour over the orange syrup and chill until ready to serve.

Preparation: 15 minutes

Cooking: 15 minutes

Serves 4 *125 calories per serving*

Selections per serving: 1½ Fruit, 50 Optional Calories

BREAD AND BUTTER PUDDING

4oz/120g bread, thinly sliced
2 tablespoons butter
3oz/90g mixed dried fruit
1½ tablespoons caster sugar
2 eggs
½ pint/300ml skimmed milk
good pinch of mixed spice

1 Spread the bread with the butter and then cut each slice into 4 triangles.

2 Arrange half of the bread, buttered side uppermost, in a 1½-pint/900ml ovenproof dish. Sprinkle half of the mixed fruit and sugar over the top.

3 Arrange the remaining bread and butter, buttered side uppermost, on top of the mixed fruit and sprinkle with the remaining fruit and sugar.

4 Whisk the eggs together with the milk and mixed spice. Pour over the bread and leave to stand for 20-30 minutes.

5 Bake in a preheated oven at 180°C/350°F/Gas Mark 4 for 30-40 minutes, until golden.

Preparation: 10 minutes plus standing time

Cooking: 30-40 minutes

Serves 4 *260 calories per serving*

Selections per serving:
1 Carbohydrate (Bread), ½ Fruit, ½ Protein, ¼ Milk, 90 Optional Calories

BAKING

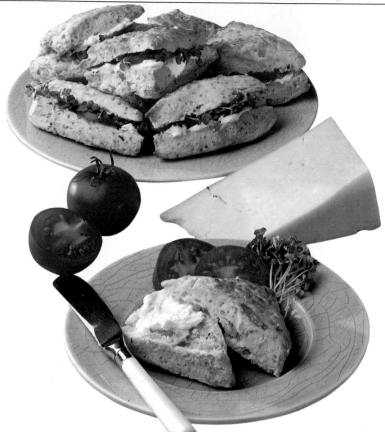

7 Mix the low-fat soft cheese and fromage frais. Add pepper sauce to taste. Serve the scones slightly warm spread with the cheese mixture, garnished with cress and tomato.

Preparation: 10 minutes

Cooking: 12-15 minutes

Serves 10 (1 scone each)
215 calories per serving

Selections per serving:
1 Carbohydrate (Bread), 1 Fat,
½ Protein, ¼ Vegetable,
30 Optional Calories

NUTTY FRUIT SQUARES

4 tablespoons margarine
4 tablespoons syrup or clear honey
2 tablespoons soft brown sugar
6oz/180g rolled oats
1oz/30g currants
1oz/30g sultanas
1oz/30g ready-to-eat dried apricots, chopped
1oz/30g flaked almonds

1 Preheat the oven to 180°C/ 350°F/Gas Mark 4.
2 Melt the margarine and syrup or honey in a saucepan. Stir in the sugar and heat gently for 2-3 minutes until dissolved.
3 Stir in the oats and add the currants, sultanas, apricots and almonds. Press into a shallow square tin and level the surface.
4 Bake in the oven for approximately 30 minutes. Cool in the tin for 5 minutes and cut into 12 pieces.

Preparation: 15 minutes

Cooking: 30 minutes

Serves 12 *155 calories per serving*

Selections per serving:
½ Carbohydrate (Bread), 1 Fat,
55 Optional Calories

CHEESE SCONES

10oz/300g plain flour
3½ teaspoons baking powder
¼ teaspoon powdered mustard
pinch of salt
4 tablespoons margarine
3oz/90g hard cheese, finely grated
2 tablespoons chopped chives
6-7fl oz/180-210ml skimmed milk
1½ teaspoons finely grated Parmesan cheese
mustard and cress
2 tomatoes, sliced
For the filling:
4oz/120g low-fat soft cheese
4oz/120g fromage frais
dash of pepper sauce

1 Line 2 baking sheets with non-stick baking parchment.
2 Reserve 1 tablespoon of flour and sift the remainder into a large bowl with the baking powder, mustard and salt. Rub the margarine into the flour.
3 Stir in the grated hard cheese and chives. Add sufficient milk to form a soft dough.
4 Sprinkle the work surface with the reserved flour and gently knead, then roll out the dough until ¾ inch/2cm thick. Cut into rounds or triangles and transfer to the baking sheets.
5 Brush the scones with a little milk and sprinkle with the Parmesan cheese. Leave at room temperature for 10 minutes.
6 Bake in a preheated oven at 210°C/425°F/Gas Mark 7 for 12-15 minutes. Cool on a wire rack.

FRESH RASPBERRY ROLL

1 teaspoon oil
3 eggs
4 tablespoons caster sugar
4oz/120g plain flour, sifted
Filling and decoration:
2 tablespoons raspberry jam
5oz/150g low-fat soft cheese
5fl oz/150ml low-fat raspberry
yogurt
5oz/150g fresh raspberries
4fl oz/120ml double cream, whipped
1 tablespoon icing sugar

1 Preheat the oven to 220°C/
425°F/Gas Mark 7.
2 Brush a 7 x 11 inch/18 x
28cm Swiss roll tin with ½ teaspoon of oil, line with greaseproof paper, and brush with the
remaining oil.
3 Whisk the eggs and sugar
until very pale and light.
4 Fold the flour lightly into the
mixture, using a metal spoon,
and pour into the prepared tin,
to cover the whole surface.
5 Bake for 7-9 minutes until
golden brown and spongy.
Meanwhile, cut out a sheet of
greaseproof paper, a little larger
than the Swiss roll tin.
6 Turn out the hot sponge on
to the paper. Peel away the lining
paper and trim the crusty edges.
Cover with a damp teatowel and
cool completely.
7 Spread the jam over the
sponge. Beat the soft cheese to
soften it and then stir in the raspberry yogurt. Add most of the
raspberries, reserving a few for
decoration. Spread over the
sponge and roll up.
8 Decorate with whipped
cream, dredge with icing sugar,
and add the reserved raspberries.

Preparation: 25 minutes

Cooking: 7-9 minutes

Serves 8 *250 calories per serving*

Selections per serving:
½ Carbohydrate (Bread),
½ Protein, 140 Optional Calories

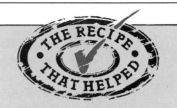

NUTTY COOKIES

As used by Carol Tanner, a
successful Weight Watchers
slimmer

3 tablespoons crunchy peanut
butter
1 tablespoon margarine
4 tablespoons golden syrup
¼ teaspoon vanilla essence
4oz/120g self-raising flour
½ teaspoon bicarbonate of soda

1 Line 2 baking sheets with
non-stick baking parchment.
2 Put the peanut butter,
margarine, golden syrup and
vanilla essence in a saucepan.
Sieve the flour and bicarbonate of soda into a bowl.
3 Gently heat the peanut
butter mixture until melted.
4 Pour the warm mixture
into the flour and mix well.
5 Roll the mixture into 12
balls and arrange on the
baking sheets. Slightly flatten
each cookie.
6 Bake at 180°C/350°F/Gas
Mark 4 for 15-20 minutes,
until light brown. Leave on
the baking sheet for 3-4
minutes and then transfer to a
cooling rack.

Preparation: 10 minutes

Cooking: 15-20 minutes

Makes 12 *85 calories per
cookie*

Selections per cookie ½ Fat,
60 Optional Calories

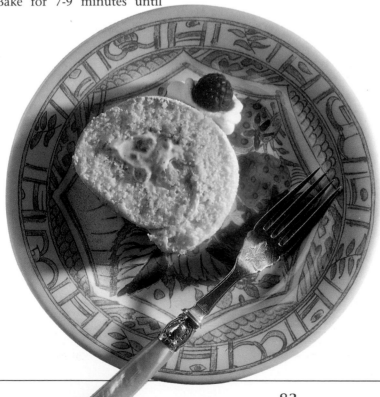

It is easy to think that dieting is all to do with the foods that you eat. Of course, the foods that you do or do not eat will have a direct influence on your weight loss or gain, but just as important is your frame of mind and the way you feel about yourself when you are dieting. If the only reason for eating food was hunger, then few of us would have a weight problem at all, but you will find that you eat for a whole host of other reasons. You may find that you eat to comfort yourself when someone upsets you or makes you angry, as a pick-me-up when you are tired or bored, as a celebration for a job well done, for a special occasion, or equally when you have allowed yourself to become over-hungry and need to feel satisfied quickly. These are the 'feelings', if you like, that make you turn to food, and it is important to realise that during your weight loss and even when you have lost weight, these feelings will still be present. They are a fact of life, and if you can learn first to identify your particular weaknesses, you will be better prepared to cope and deal with these feelings in the future, without turning to food.

It is not 'wrong' to enjoy the pleasurable sensations that eating can bring, but this new way of eating will be a stimulating challenge for you to pursue. You will be amazed to find that there is a whole host of new foods, tastes and textures waiting for you to enjoy, and, as you lose weight, how you feel about food and yourself will change.

Why did I overeat?

This question is often asked by dieters. Once you have decided to lose weight and you achieve success, you will probably ask yourself this question many times. As we have discussed before, in order to gain weight you need to eat more calories than your body requires, and in fact you need to eat 3,500 extra calories for every pound that you gain. Those extra calories have probably been added to your daily eating pattern slowly, but surely, thereby increasing your weight, pound by disheartening pound, over a period of time. It's a good idea to ask yourself just how long it has taken you to increase your weight to its present level. This will help you not to become too impatient with your slow but steady weight loss as you follow the Weight Watchers Programme.

To find out whether or not you are an emotional eater answer yes or no to the following questions. Try to be honest with yourself.

1 Do you find yourself thinking of food when you are bored?

2 Do you find that you reward yourself with food for jobs done or tasks completed, i.e. a cup of coffee and a biscuit after doing the housework, a chocolate bar when the children are tucked up in bed, or perhaps a few drinks at the end of a hard day at work?

3 Do you turn to food when people make you angry?

4 If you have stopped smoking, do you find that you have substituted food for cigarettes?

5 Does the smell of fresh bread from the supermarket persuade you to buy that hot loaf from the bakery?

6 Do you find yourself suggesting a meal out to celebrate at every possible opportunity?

The more times that you have answered 'yes', then the more likely you are to be emotionally dependent on food. Once you have identified your

CAROL TANNER

Carol Tanner used to overdose on sweets and cakes before joining Weight Watchers and losing six stone. "I used to buy cakes for the whole family and then scoff the lot. When I went on a binge I'd get so desperate, after eating the cupboards bare I would then start on gâteaux straight from the freezer!"

Being at home with two young children and getting depressed about her weight left Carol seeking solace in the biscuit barrel. "I felt happy when I was eating, although I hardly tasted the mounds of food. Afterwards I would feel so terrible. I would hide food so I could eat it secretly, and then tell my husband that I couldn't understand why I was putting on weight; after all, I hardly ate a thing!"

At husband Chris's Christmas party at work, Carol couldn't even squeeze into a size 24 dress, and the final straw came when Chris booked a holiday to Ibiza. Carol was filled with terror at the prospect of stripping off on the beach, and she decided to join Weight Watchers. 'I desperately wanted to lose weight, but I was very shy and worried about joining on my own."

However, Carol enthusiastically set about working her way down to her Goal Weight of 10 stone. "Some weeks I didn't lose any weight, and that was disheartening. Then I started to measure myself too – each week I found that I was slimmer even if I wasn't lighter. It took me six months to reach my goal. I felt like shouting the news from the rooftops."

Carol now says that her whole personality has changed. "By that I mean that I now actually have a personality. I'm a lot more forward instead of hiding behind my husband all the time. All my life I've dreamed of being slim. Now I look forward to going out, talking to people and just getting my fair share of the attention at last." By sticking to her healthy eating habits, Carol has managed to maintain her slim figure. Gone is the insatiable sweet tooth and the lack of confidence that made her reluctant to leave the sanctuary of her home. She now lives life to the full and her husband says that he has fallen in love all over again 'with a new woman!'

STATISTICS: CAROL	
AGE:	35
HEIGHT:	5 feet 6 inches
WAS:	16 stone
NOW:	10 stone
LOST:	6 stone

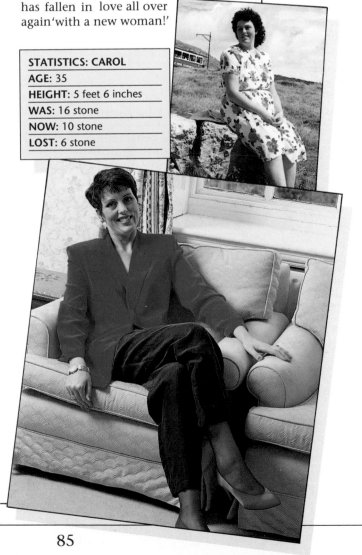

particular weakness, then you need to set up plans to conquer those specific situations that cause you to turn to food as a comfort or emotional prop. The following suggestions may help you. Try them out for yourself.

● When you are bored, divert your attention to jobs that need doing, or use this time to take up a new hobby or pastime

● Instead of rewarding yourself with food after a task well done, treat yourself instead with a favourite magazine or beauty treatment or a chat with a friend, either in person or on the phone

● When you are angry, ask yourself if that piece of cake or biscuit will really help make you less so. The cake will take only seconds to eat but will set your dieting plans back far further

● If you have stopped smoking, satisfy your need for oral gratification with low-calorie peppermints, sugar-free chewing gum or small cubes of raw vegetables – not high-calorie snacks

● Try to do your food shopping just after you have eaten a meal – never shop when you are hungry

● Always prepare a shopping list before you visit the supermarket. Some of the aisles can be missed completely and the chances are that the aroma of freshly baked bread is merely a chemical in the ventilation system designed to lure you to the bakery counter!

● By all means enjoy a celebratory meal whenever you wish, but plan your indulgences. If you do go overboard, get back on the track at the very next meal and start over. Don't dwell on the past

Learning to overcome these situations really is possible. You *can* do it,

you need not be dependent on food for comfort, and eventually you will feel confident enough to say 'no' easily in times of difficulty.

I feel deprived

'Why me?' is often the cry of many a dieter. It can sometimes be hard to understand why it is necessary for you to diet when all around you are apparently eating to their hearts' content and never gaining a pound. We all have slender, sylph-like friends who eat endless amounts of chocolate, enjoy chips with every meal, exercise rarely and yet have figures that make them eligible for the pages of *Vogue* magazine. Life can sometimes seem unfair, but if you can only accept that we are not all the same, you will be able to stop feeling sorry for yourself and just accept that the task ahead is both achievable and bearable.

Feeling sorry for yourself is really another emotion that will drive you to food for comfort. If you feel miserable and deprived, the chances are that you will develop the 'what does it matter anyway' attitude. This will drive you to food, with the result that you will again feel miserable and the vicious cycle is repeated.

When you next feel deprived, *stop*. Ask yourself exactly why you feel this way. Is it the situation you're in? Think carefully before you eat in haste. Remember, no foods are forbidden on the Weight Watchers Programme, so if you are feeling deprived and the temptation isn't too great, why not enjoy 'a little of what you fancy' – staying in control of how much you eat. Account for the calories and feel good that you are in control. If, however, the temptation is too great and you cannot cope with small amounts of this yearned-for treat, then employ avoidance tactics! Move away from the temptation and occupy yourself elsewhere until the craving has passed.

There really is no need to feel sorry for yourself. As the new you emerges, those feelings will pale into insignificance when stacked against the feelings of pure delight that await you and your new shape.

Hang on in there!

You have probably wondered how long it will take for you to achieve your target weight. Have you already set yourself a goal of how much you should lose by a particular date? If you have, then the chances are that you will be disappointed. Slowly but surely is the answer. If you learn to take your weight loss slowly, pound by pound, you are less likely to fail. The sooner you accept the fact that you must take each day as it comes, the easier your diet will become. Make it your aim to be successful for one day at a time. On some days, when the going gets tough, you may have to take one hour at a time, but one thing you can be sure of – you *will* succeed if you hang on in there.

Don't make excuses!

There are probably lots of reasons that you can think of for not losing weight. Here are just a few of the most common excuses given by dieters. Do you recognise any of them? Are they your own excuses?

- I've got a low metabolic rate
- I am genetically meant to be overweight
- I have large bones; this is not really excessive weight that I am carrying
- I have some difficult social occasions on the horizon. I will start my diet after these have passed
- I hardly eat enough to keep a fly alive. I don't understand why I am overweight
- I have a problem with my glands
- I suffer from fluid retention
- My hormones make me overweight
- I am addicted to chocolate (of course, this could be cheese, bread or anything else for that matter!)
- I need more food because I have an active lifestyle
- I have no willpower
- I eat far less than the rest of my family. I cannot understand why I am the only one with a weight problem
- I cannot lose weight in the summer (of course, this could be spring, winter, autumn or all four seasons!)
- My partner likes me the way I am.
- I don't want to lose weight. I'm happy the way I am

All of these are excuses, except the last. If you really don't want to change, then don't diet. When you have decided that you *can* diet, here are some familiar excuses that you may try and use when you want to eat those foods that you know you should avoid.

1 This little bit won't hurt.
2 Food eaten when you are standing up doesn't count.
3 Food eaten secretly contains no calories.
4 Diet soft drinks counteract the calories of chocolate.
5 Alcohol is OK when diluted with low-calorie mixers.

How do I feel?

6 This skirt won't fit me because it has shrunk at the cleaners.

7 What I am experiencing is middle-aged spread. All women/men of my age expect to be heavier during these years.

All of the above are excuses and bear no resemblance to the truth.

The Weight Watchers Programme has been created by nutritional experts. There is absolutely no shadow of a doubt, if you follow the Programme to the letter, that you will succeed. All of the above excuses are just that – excuses! Follow the Programme, think positively and watch the weight disappear. Your need for excuses will diminish as your diet progresses, but be reassured that the excuses that you have made have been expressed by many dieters before you. You are not alone but only you can take control of your own destiny. If you want to succeed you will. The success stories in this book bear testimony to this.

I've reached a weight loss plateau – help!

It's a well known fact that everyone loses weight at a different pace. After the initial spurt during the first stages of your diet, you will find that your average weight loss settles down at a steady one or two pounds each week. However, the word 'average' is very important. You may well find that some weeks you will lose more than this amount and some weeks less. There may even be short spells when you lose nothing at all. This stage is known as a weight loss plateau and can be quite a challenge to any dieter.

In practical terms, what happens to your body during this stage is that tem-porarily the scales do not register a weight loss. You may well think you are following the Programme to the letter, but are you really sure that the odd snack now and again isn't creeping into your everyday eating plans? Are you sure you are not eating more food than you readily admit? Remember how at the beginning of your diet we asked you to weigh and measure all of your foods. Perhaps that 1oz slice of bread that you enjoyed with breakfast today was actually closer to 2oz or even 3oz. In isolation, this isn't a problem but build this up over a week and it's easy to see how your weight loss efforts can be jeopardized.

As mentioned in the exercise section on page 96, exercising regularly will help you to burn off excess calories, and long term will increase your metabolic rate. Hand on heart, how much exercise have you done this past week? When weight loss temporarily stops, this is the cue to make a determined effort to incorporate exercise once again into your daily routine.

However, it may be that you have stuck to the diet and exercised and still your weight loss has stopped. If this is the case, *don't panic*.

Sometimes this does happen. Your body is taking a temporary rest from those unwanted pounds and may even be retaining more fluid than usual, hence the apparent 'marking time' phenomenon. If you just continue to take one day at a time your rewards will soon register once again on the scales. If you panic you are likely to go off the rails and possibly undo all the good work of recent weeks. Use the easy checklist on page 90 to find the tactics you need to employ to conquer this temporary psychological set-back.

88

MORVEN BURR

Since losing over five stone, Morven Burr has become much more out-going and self-confident. "When I was fat, there were a lot of things I would have liked to have done but I was scared what people would think of me. However, I now wear and do whatever I want and don't feel that I have to hide in a corner because I'm so fat. In fact, I feel years younger."

Morven put on weight during her three pregnancies. She had her children close together and never lost the excess weight she was carrying. Before joining Weight Watchers, she tried various diets, but none of them worked. "When the weather was warm or when I had to hurry, I became short of breath. Even changing the babies' nappies was a struggle!"

When she joined Weight Watchers, Morven changed her eating habits for good. "The Programme is easy to follow, and you can still allow yourself occasional treats. I have learned how to eat a healthy, enjoyable diet which will keep off those unwanted extra pounds."

Morven used to get discouraged when she felt that she had had a 'good' week but the scales didn't reflect this. "However, after several weeks of attending Meetings, I noticed that if my weight stuck or went up one week, the next week I had a good weight loss, so I persevered. Everyone was very supportive, and talking to my Leader and the other Members helped."

Morven's life has been transformed since reaching her Goal Weight. "I enjoy going out a lot more and wearing flattering clothes. I've joined an aerobics class and go disco dancing. In the past, it was always my husband who took the children swimming, but now I don't mind baring my body in the water!"

She has even started a youth club for mentally handicapped youngsters, and takes part in all their sporting activities. "I would have just supervised them before I lost weight, but now I ski, swim, trampoline, quad bike and even play football with them." Eating a healthy diet, exercising regularly and staying slim are now second nature to Morven, and she is determined to keep it that way.

STATISTICS: MORVEN	
AGE:	29
HEIGHT:	5 feet 4 inches
WAS:	14 stone 12½ pounds
NOW:	9 stone 7½ pounds
LOST:	5 stone 5 pounds

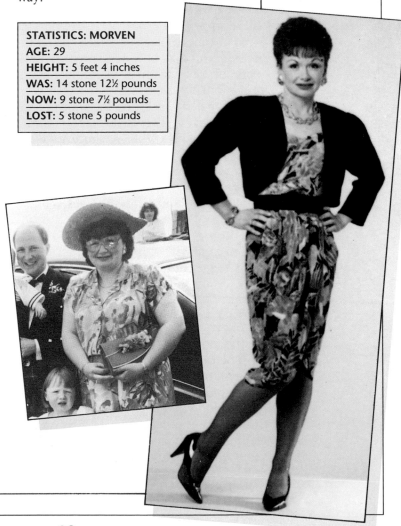

Weight loss plateau checklist

1 Plan your meals in advance so that you have a set plan of action for the coming days of the week.

2 Weigh and measure your food again for one complete week.

3 Plan to exercise at least twice this week if this is not usually part of your routine.

4 Instead of weighing yourself this week, measure yourself; although your weight loss may have stopped, the tape measure will show that those inches are still disappearing.

5 For women: keep a track of your periods; you may be able to identify patterns in your weight loss connected to your monthly cycle.

6 Jot down five reasons for wanting to lose weight in the first place - these reasons will give you the incentive to continue.

A weight loss plateau is not the end of the world; it is just a way for your body to take stock, and adjust to your weight loss so far. Don't despair! You will soon start losing again, and you'll be better able to cope with this situation should it happen again in the future.

Hey! I feel slimmer!

As the pounds disappear, it won't be long before you really do feel slimmer. You will be gaining confidence, perhaps wearing clothes a size smaller and really feeling good about yourself. Now is the time to take advantage of this slight feeling of euphoria. Why not treat yourself to a luxurious beauty routine or article of clothing to flatter the emerging new you?

Fashion to flatter you

Part of the pleasure of looking good and feeling good is wearing new clothes and fashions that are flattering, and most people who join Weight Watchers confess that one of their main reasons for slimming is to be able to wear the clothes they like – instead of the limited range that is available in the larger sizes. Few of us can afford a new wardrobe every time we lose half a stone, but that doesn't mean to say we should wait until we reach our target weight to change the way we dress. Nothing gives a bigger boost to our confidence than making the most of a new slimmer figure! The first thing you should do is to get the proportions right.

● Never wear clothes that stop at your widest point, because that draws the eye immediately. Go for neutral-coloured dresses without fussy detail, and long, softly tailored jackets that skim the hips

● Choose slim-line skirts that reach over the knee, in a dark plain colour. Avoid multi-coloured prints with big brash patterns and gathered or layered skirts; they can make even slim people look tubby

● For casual wear, you can't do better than to buy yourself a pair of stretch leggings in black or navy and some big, bright, baggy T-shirts or sloppy shirts; it's a look that suits all sizes

● Emphasise your good points. Make pretty legs look longer by wearing heels, but avoid thin straps at the ankles, which make legs look bigger

● Discreet shoulder pads and a long-line jacket will give you a slimmer look. A pretty scarf draped softly around your shoulders will have the same effect

MICHAEL RYAN

Since joining Weight Watchers, Michael Ryan has managed to lose an amazing 114 pounds to achieve his Goal Weight of 11 stone 7 pounds. He had been overweight for 15 years and says, "I was just eating too much of the wrong kinds of food, such as biscuits, chocolate and take-away meals. Giving up smoking 10 years ago didn't help matters either."

As a hotelier, Michael is in a job where weight gain is generally regarded as an occupational hazard, and before he joined Weight Watchers he had tried all sorts of diets without any success. The birth of his son gave him the incentive he needed to go along to his local Meeting. At first, only his wife knew that he had joined, but when his weight loss became noticeable, he told people the secret of his success. "Usually their reaction was one of surprise: 'Do men go to Weight Watchers?' People who don't have a weight problem can't really understand how difficult it is to lose weight, but the support and encourage-

ment of my Leader and fellow Members helped me to succeed."

Michael never felt discouraged, although he admits that it was difficult sometimes to say 'No' to temptation. "When I was tempted to eat more of something, I'd ask myself, 'What do you really want to do: eat more or be slim?' I usually overcame my desire to eat!"

His whole family has benefited from the change in his eating habits. "My son eats very few sweet things because he doesn't see me eat them very often. Now he likes to join me in eating an apple. My wife also eats more healthily. Also, I have more energy to enjoy my family."

Michael's whole life has changed. He works out at a local gym and he has more confidence and energy at work. "In the past, I didn't want to be noticed and I lacked confidence when meeting new people. Now I enjoy going out as often as I can. I have more peace of mind and my health has improved." Michael is determined to stay slim and give his children a healthy future.

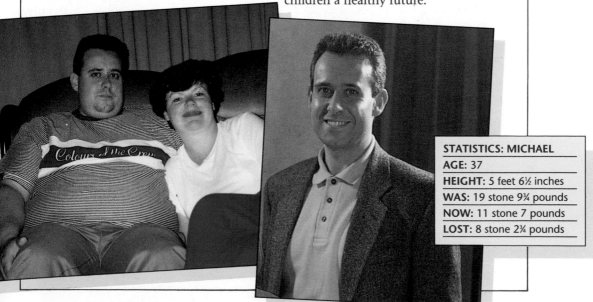

STATISTICS: MICHAEL
AGE: 37
HEIGHT: 5 feet 6½ inches
WAS: 19 stone 9¾ pounds
NOW: 11 stone 7 pounds
LOST: 8 stone 2¾ pounds

SUE CALLAWAY

Sue's weight problem was caused not so much by her love of food, but by her lack of self-confidence, which stood in the way of a slim body. "I suddenly realised that my weight was a defence mechanism. I didn't think too much of myself, so I thought that if I stayed fat nobody would bother with me." However, the day came when Sue weighed herself and reached her lowest point. "I was disgusted with myself for weighing nearly 14 stone and having to buy size 18 clothes. Before, I'd hide my sadness beneath a smile, but I just couldn't pretend any more."

Sue enrolled at Weight Watchers. "When they gave me my Goal Weight of 10 stone I thought, 'I'll never get to that!' I had to completely change my eating habits. I've never eaten because I'm hungry; it was always just something to do. It was all the wrong type of food too – biscuits and crisps." and everything went smoothly until she hit a weight loss plateau. "The weight just wouldn't move. I felt like giving up, but I stuck at it. Then something clicked and I lost the weight quite quickly."

Sue can now feel doubly proud of her achievement – she has lost weight and kept it off successfully. She now loves going out dancing with her friends, and even to aerobics twice a week. She is no longer too self-conscious to talk to people, and is determined to do all the things she's always dreamed of. "I want to live and enjoy life to the full. I'm learning to drive and another goal I want to achieve is to work in a hotel, so I can meet new people. Now the weight has gone, this is me – for all to see!"

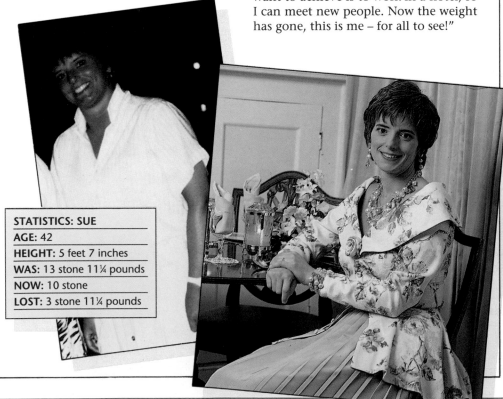

STATISTICS: SUE

AGE:	42
HEIGHT:	5 feet 7 inches
WAS:	13 stone 11¼ pounds
NOW:	10 stone
LOST:	3 stone 11¼ pounds

● Choose scooped or boat necks if your neck is short and plump. V-necks give a longer slimmer line to any bodice

● Avoid safari-type jackets, or shirts and blouses with pockets on the bust which will make you look bulky; and never be tempted to buy shiny, tightly fitting evening wear. Stick to cool and classic looks. Remember that a 'little black dress' is always elegant and flattering and never dates

● Although black is one of the most flattering and slimming colours you can choose, make it smart and not drab; overweight people are used to dressing to be ignored, and as you lose weight you can afford to dress to be noticed. Wearing bright colours can really brighten your mood!

● Avoid puffed sleeves that make you look wider in the upper body

● Rather than wear a tightly fitting tailored jacket, choose a flowing, floppy jacket in a soft natural fabric such as cotton, linen or silk which will hang loosely and create a flattering triangular silhouette

Won't it cost the earth?

If your clothes are just falling off you, of course you'll need to replenish at least the basics in your wardrobe – but it needn't cost the earth. Choose softly fitting clothes rather than the strictly tailored look, so that you can still wear them when you've lost more weight.

Snip and tuck

If you're handy with the sewing machine, or have a mum or a friend who is, your old clothes can be altered

Fashion tips for men
The same rules apply for men: don't wear garish colours as these will draw attention to your shape; and don't wear horizontal stripes. Vertical stripes will elongate and are more slimming. Try wearing braces instead of belts; they take the focus away from the waistline.

with darts and tucks to fit the new slimmer-line you. Alternatively, look in the local paper or scan notice-board ads for a dressmaker who's willing to undertake alterations cheaply.

Second-hand

It's amazing how many shops there are nowadays selling good-quality used clothes. With a little patience you can find great bargains; it might be a good opportunity to get rid of all those clothes you've 'slimmed out of'!

Accessorize!

Another cheap way of updating your wardrobe while you're losing weight is to buy yourself some stylish and fashionable accessories. Use them to dress up an outfit, or ring the changes for different occasions.

● Shawls and scarves, held in place with a brooch, can draw the eye away from heavy hips, and flattering colours can enhance those of your lips and eyes. Try throwing a bright shawl in fine thin cotton or wool across one shoulder

● Go for bold dramatic earrings rather than delicate 'droppers', and wear long chunky necklaces for a more slimming line. Avoid tight chokers and ankle chains

● Choose wide belts that emphasise your waist as you slim down, but don't cinch them in too tightly.

A hairstyle to flatter you

Now that you're starting to lose weight, it's time to take a good look at your hair. Why not choose a new, more flattering style? A good hairstyle can make you look slimmer by making your neck and face look longer, and you'll feel better if you get rid of split ends and give your hair a healthy shine too.

Sometimes it takes a lot of courage to change your hairstyle radically, and you may find it easier to make any changes to the cut or colour only gradually over the course of several visits to the hairdresser. Choose a style that not only suits you, but also your hair type and which is suitable for your lifestyle. There is no point opting for a complex style that requires extra care when washing and setting, and frequent cuts, if you don't have the time for this. Choose something more manageable instead. Remember that highlights or a subtle change of colour can also help to create a new look.

Keep your hair in tip-top condition by using conditioners, protein packs and hot oil treatments.

Styles that flatter

● If you have a square face, go for a soft look of medium- or shoulder-length hair with waves falling sideways over your shoulders

● If you have a round, full face, wear your hair long or choose a shorter style with narrower lines

● If your face is oblong, make it appear wider with a waving frame of medium-length hair, which is full at the sides

● A short, soft feathery style that's easy to maintain is often a good option while you're still losing weight. Avoid heavy fringes and locks that straggle onto your collar, and note that hair that's tightly pulled back or severely crew cut will make your face look fuller.

What make-up should I use?

Make-up, like jewellery, can be used to dramatic effect, and can draw the eye to your best features. The latest look is fresh and natural – not heavy.

● Apply foundation and blusher *sparingly*, using the blusher to delicately slim your face by emphasising your cheek bones. Powder lightly for a smooth, velvety finish. Use a concealer cream or stick to cover up spots or blemishes, or to disguise dark rings under the eyes

● To make small eyes look larger, apply some dark shadow along the socket line and a paler shadow on the lids

● To make eyes look more widely spaced, brush pale highlighter on the skin on either side of the bridge of your nose, and apply a dark triangle of shadow to the outer corners of the upper eyelids

● You can make thin lips look fuller by outlining them just outside their natural line and then filling in with lipstick

● To make full lips appear less prominent, draw a line just *inside* your natural lipline with a lighter lipstick, and then fill in with a darker colour

● Why not treat yourself to a make over? This is a wonderful chance to try out new colours and get professional tips on showing off your best features

JANET AND PETER GARSDEN-COOPER

In 1976, Janet Garsden-Cooper won the title Miss British Isles, but 10 years later she was overweight and unhappy. She failed to regain her slim figure after the birth of her baby, and then separation and divorce from her first husband meant that she was leading a very stressful life as a single working parent.

"Stress led to bad eating habits and comfort eating," says Jan. "Most of my nicer clothes wouldn't fit me. I felt ugly, lumpy and frumpish. I also felt tired and became breathless after any effort. I didn't want to meet new people, knowing they would see me as a fatty."

But then Janet met the new man in her life and together they enrolled at Weight Watchers. "I knew that my fiancé was reluctant to set our wedding date until we had both lost weight, and that made me determined." She was also encouraged by her friends, one of whom took a video ("It shows my bottom wobbling in a pink track suit – horrible" and threatened to play it back if she didn't reach her target weight.

It worked. Jan found that Weight Watchers provided her with a varied balanced diet with no forbidden foods. "I was able to have a little chocolate and alcohol, and still remain on the Programme and lose weight."

Both Jan and Peter, now her husband, succeeded, and now the whole family enjoys a healthier way of eating, especially salads, fruit and natural yogurt. What's more, Jan looks as glamorous as she did on the day when she won Miss British Isles. She loves to dress classically in clothes that mix and match, choosing black, grey, red and cream for a superbly elegant wardrobe. However, when she was a stone heavier, she used to hide her shape by dressing in baggy clothes and tracksuits.

Jan says: "I went to Weight Watchers on the morning of my wedding day. I had reached my goal. I wore my gold pin on my wedding dress!" No wonder Jan was chosen as Weight Watchers Fashion Ambassador of the Year for 1992-93.

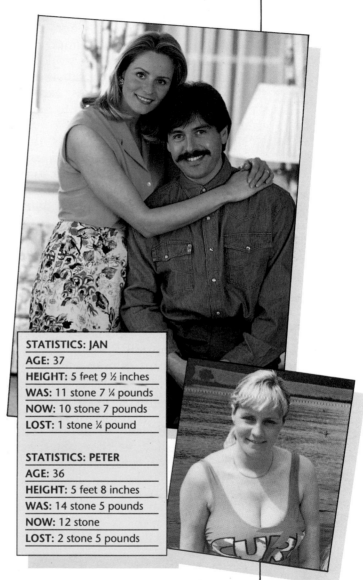

STATISTICS: JAN	
AGE:	37
HEIGHT:	5 feet 9 ½ inches
WAS:	11 stone 7 ¼ pounds
NOW:	10 stone 7 pounds
LOST:	1 stone ¼ pound

STATISTICS: PETER	
AGE:	36
HEIGHT:	5 feet 8 inches
WAS:	14 stone 5 pounds
NOW:	12 stone
LOST:	2 stone 5 pounds

E
xercise will help speed up your weight loss and tone up your body to improve your new shape. With this in mind, we have created a special home work-out programme to get you started. It has been devised by our fitness expert, Derrick Evans, and is designed to make exercising enjoyable and fun.

The problem with exercise is that sometimes it doesn't sound like fun, and if you are trying to break a life-long habit of *not* exercising, it can seem particularly daunting. However, don't despair. It's never too late to start exercising, and it will bring very tangible results and benefits.

Why exercise?

You may ask yourself: 'Why should I bother exercising?' – especially if you are losing weight steadily. Well, exercise not only burns up calories and helps you to lose weight faster, and makes you feel fitter and healthier. It also helps to curb your appetite so that it is easier for you to follow our Programme. Regular exercise, say three times a week, will bring the following benefits:

● It will firm up and tone stubborn problem areas such as the stomach, bottom, hips and thighs

● It will strengthen your muscles and make you look slimmer

● It will raise your energy level

● It will help you to beat the stress in your life. Scientific research shows that people who exercise regularly are three times more likely to relax when under stress

● It will help make your heart and lungs work more efficiently and improve your circulation

● It will improve your posture and flexibility so that you walk taller and look slimmer

However, in spite of all the obvious advantages that exercise can bring, there are still many people who have not taken the plunge, so why don't they exercise?

Excuses! Excuses!

Some of the most common reasons for not exercising go like this:

● "I don't have the time."

● "I don't like exercise."

● "I'm too old!"

● "I can't afford it."

● "There's nowhere to go. There's no gym or leisure centre nearby."

● "I'm going to wait until I lose some weight."

Do any of these excuses sound familiar to you? Are they ones that you use yourself? However, they don't stand up to close examination. We can all make the time to do some exercise – just 10 minutes a day will get you off to a good start. If you don't exercise, how do you know if you like it or not? If you choose the right sort for you, it will be enjoyable and fun.

You don't necessarily need special

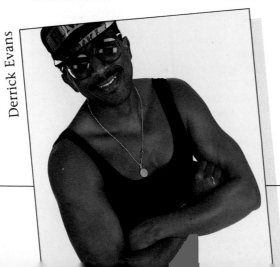

Derrick Evans

LINZI LLOYD-HENRY

Looking at Linzi now with her 'model' looks, it is difficult to believe that before she joined Weight Watchers she was three stone heavier. Linzi had always been overweight, and had spent most of her adult life on the relentless treadmill of crash diets, followed by weight gain. She confesses, "I've done them all – anything that came out! But they just don't work, especially the meal replacements. Once you start to eat food again, you revert back to how you were." Linzi used to snack between meals on biscuits and nuts but they did not satisfy her hunger, and she would still eat large meals.

At last, on a family holiday, when Linzi realised that she must brave the swimming pool or deprive her little girl of her holiday fun, she decided to really do something about her weight. She now laughs at her initial reservations about joining Weight Watchers. "I was worried about what it would be like. I felt a bit self-conscious, but I went with my friend and discovered my fears were unfounded."

When she had lost one stone, Linzi started back on the road to fitness by joining a local gym, and she has not looked back since: "I do an average three to four hours of aerobics a week. I can't get enough of it."

Linzi now eats regular meals and works out in her local aerobics class several times a week to tone up her new figure and stay slim. She enjoys exercise so much she has recently taken part in an aerobics challenge which she would never have dreamed of before. She thinks that her success is due to combining her diet with regular exercise, and that this is the key to effective weight loss.

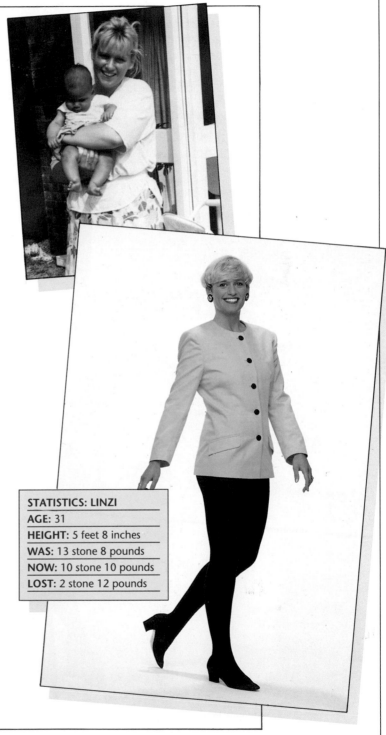

STATISTICS: LINZI	
AGE:	31
HEIGHT:	5 feet 8 inches
WAS:	13 stone 8 pounds
NOW:	10 stone 10 pounds
LOST:	2 stone 12 pounds

facilities nearby. You can walk, jog, cycle or do our home work-out programme; you can do these anywhere at any time and they don't cost anything.

You are never too old to start exercising, if you do it gradually and sensibly. As you get older, you may not have the suppleness and strength of a younger person, but you can still keep yourself fit. Do some gentle stretching exercises to start you off and help improve your flexibility. Some gyms and leisure centres run special exercise classes for the over-50s or over-60s, where the exercises are carefully monitored.

Start now! Don't wait until you reach your target weight before you start exercising. If you feel self-conscious you can always work out at home. As you get slimmer and more confident, you can

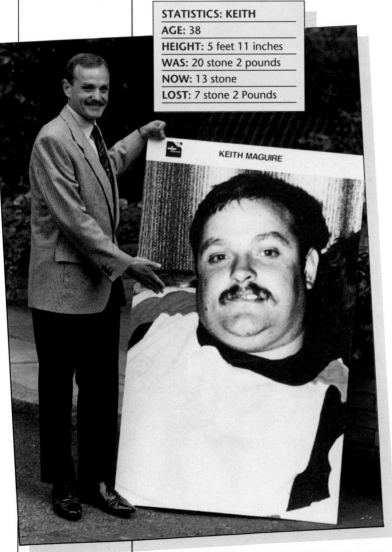

STATISTICS: KEITH	
AGE:	38
HEIGHT:	5 feet 11 inches
WAS:	20 stone 2 pounds
NOW:	13 stone
LOST:	7 stone 2 Pounds

KEITH MAGUIRE

KEITH MAGUIRE

Exercise and sport now play a big part in Keith Maguire's life, but it wasn't always like that. Before he took the decision to join Weight Watchers, he never exercised at all and suffered from shortage of breath and chest pains.

He went along to his local Meeting with his wife, and they helped each other to lose weight. It took Keith nearly a year to lose a momentous 7 stone but it was well worth it. His wife and children are proud of his achievement, and they are all eating a healthier diet.

One of the biggest changes in Keith's life since losing weight is a better social life. "We have now started to do a lot more, and enjoy a visit to the theatre, a pleasant walk and other outdoor activities instead of just a meal and drinks. I am able to do a lot more with my family. I have far more energy and can keep up with my nine-year-old twin boys."

Keith can now join in the exercise he enjoys and be a more active, energetic father to his sons. He has not experienced any difficulties in maintaining his weight now that he has changed his lifestyle and eating habits. He feels confident that he can cope with anything.

venture outside and take up jogging or join an exercise class.

How do I start?

If you want to start exercising, it is important not to rush in and overdo it as this may lead to injury and disappointment. You don't have to 'go for the burn' or feel physically exhausted afterwards for exercise to do you good. You don't have to run thirty miles a week or spend hours exercising to attain a good level of fitness. Exercise should be fun and energizing – you should always finish feeling as though you could do a little more, not completely exhausted.

So what is an acceptable level of activity which will benefit you and help you to lose weight? Experts think that exercising just three times a week for twenty to thirty minutes will do you good and make you fitter. There are lots of ways in which you can increase your activity and burn up more calories. Look at the box and try out some of our suggestions.

When you select a new exercise regime, always look for the 'enjoyment factor'. If you enjoy doing it, you will stick with it and make it a permanent part of your life. Ideally, the sort of exercise you choose should tone up your body, build your strength, and increase your flexibility and stamina. It should also be convenient in terms of accessibility and timing, so why not try out one of the following?

1 Aerobics or exercise class
2 Ball and racket sports
3 Bowling
4 Cycling
5 Golf
6 Jogging or running
7 Judo, karate or tai chi
8 Swimming and water aerobics
9 Team games

Increase your activity

- Always walk up the stairs rather than taking the lift or escalator
- Try to walk rather than drive at every available opportunity
- Go for a walk during your lunch break
- Get off the bus one stop earlier and walk the rest of the way
- Park your car further away and walk to the office or shops
- Take your dog for a walk
- Go for a family walk in the park or a cycle ride in the country at weekends
- Buy an exercise bike or rowing machine
- Dust off your bike and hit the road
- Take up a new sport, e.g. badminton, jogging, swimming, dancing or aerobics
- Join an exercise class
- Work out at home

10 Walking
11 Weight training
12 Yoga

Walking

Walking is the easiest exercise of all – and it costs nothing. It is very gentle and you are less likely to suffer from any stiffness, muscle soreness or injuries than in other physical activities, such as jogging. You can walk at any time and make it part of your daily routine. Make sure that you wear sensible shoes; flat, comfortable ones that provide support.

Try to walk as many times a week as possible, preferably every day. Walk for at least twenty to thirty minutes, aiming to cover as much distance as possible. As you get fitter, you will find that you can walk further more quickly. It is a good idea to work out a circuit from your home and time yourself each day.

How you walk is also important. Hold your stomach in, with your shoulders, head and neck held high. Keep your elbows and arms close to your body. They should be bent and relaxed – not tense or held awkwardly. Walk briskly, breathing deeply.

Jogging

If you are unused to exercise, it is best to start off very slowly with a combination of jogging and walking. For example, work out a short circuit round your local streets or park and then alternate walking and jogging by walking briskly to one lamp post or tree and then jogging to the next. Give yourself sufficient time to recover between the spurts of jogging. As you get fitter, you will gradually start to jog more and walk less. Here are some tips to get you going:

● Run on grass rather than on the road or pavements

● Don't run on your toes – push off with the ball of your foot

● Keep your arms bent and relaxed at your sides

● Invest in a good pair of training shoes

● Wear loose, comfortable clothing

● Always run where it's safe to do so; don't take risks!

Cycling

If you are thinking of getting your bike out and cycling to get fit, check it over first to make sure that the brakes and lights are working properly. You should wear a helmet, and some reflective strips on your clothing if you cycle at night.

To get the maximum benefit, you should choose a route that combines flat stretches with uphill and downhill ones.

You could even make cycling a family activity.

Swimming

This is one of the best forms of exercise because it tones and streamlines your whole body. It is also very safe and particularly good for people with muscle injuries or joint problems. Try to do a variety of strokes.

Exercise guidelines and safety code

Before you rush off to exercise, read this section carefully. There are always risks with any form of exercise but if you do it sensibly and correctly, you will minimize these and can only benefit.

● **Consult your doctor:** He will help by advising on which activity is best for you. You must be sure to do this if you smoke or drink heavily or have a medical condition, chest pains, heart disease, high blood pressure, tender or painful joints, any other illnesses or are pregnant

● **Always warm-up:** You should do this gently with a few stretching exercises (see page 104) before you start

● **Begin very gently:** Increase the frequency and intensity gradually. Build up the number of exercises and repetitions slowly

● **Do not strain:** Stretch only as far as feels comfortable

● **Listen to your body:** It will always tell you when the going is getting too tough – or too easy

● **Don't exercise after a meal:** It is better to exercise before eating

● **Vary the exercise:** This will stop it becoming boring and you giving up

DENISE STEELE

Looking at Denise now, it's hard to believe that she weighed over 17 stone before she embarked on the Weight Watchers Programme. For Denise has slimmed from a size 24 to a size 12, and there is no longer any need to hide her body away under baggy clothes. "I wore long plain skirts because that was all I could find to fit over my huge legs and hips. I hated my appearance so much."

For years, Denise had overeaten. "I used to have a big cooked breakfast, and then on the way to school I'd stop off at the bakery and buy sausage rolls and doughnuts. At lunchtime I ate my packed lunch plus a school dinner, then finished off with crisps. Walking home from school I would buy more doughnuts, and continue to eat non-stop until dinner time when I was too full to eat a proper meal."

The holiday photos of a trip to Canada and seeing a Weight Watchers advertisement on TV spurred Denise into joining Weight Watchers. She was worried initially about whether she would be allowed enough food to prevent her feeling hungry, but, as she discovered, "There's plenty to eat on the Programme, and it's simple to follow. For the first time in my life I realised how tasty vegetables and fruit are!"

It took sixteen months for Denise to reach her Goal Weight but she persevered, and it was well worth the effort. Not only did she lose weight but she also started exercising to tone up her body. "My mum, who joined Weight Watchers with me, had started jogging to get fit. As she loved it so much, I thought I'd try it too, but I found it a chore. Instead of giving up totally on fitness though, I decided to try aerobics, and I couldn't get enough of it! The

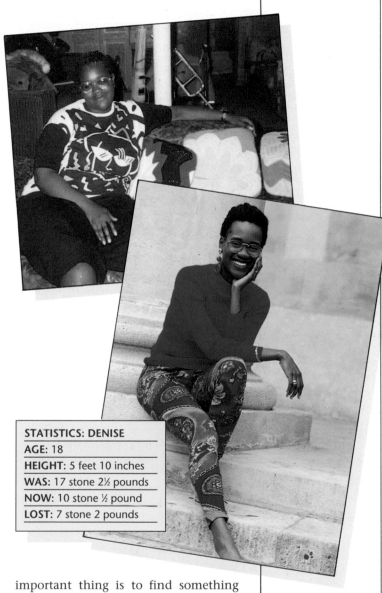

STATISTICS: DENISE	
AGE: 18	
HEIGHT: 5 feet 10 inches	
WAS: 17 stone 2½ pounds	
NOW: 10 stone ½ pound	
LOST: 7 stone 2 pounds	

important thing is to find something you enjoy doing and then you'll want to keep on going."

Now Denise not only goes to aerobics classes but she also swims and tap dances – all the things she felt too self-conscious to do when she was overweight.

● **Set aside time:** Plan your exercise, making some time each day if possible

● **Exercise with a friend:** You may encourage and motivate each other

● **Stop if you feel pain:** If you experience pain, dizziness or generally feel unwell, stop immediately. If the symptoms persist, consult your doctor

● **Cool down afterwards:** Do this with some gentle stretching exercises to ease out your muscles (see page 116).

Breathe deeply

Breathing correctly while you exercise will help you to be more aware of your body and perform the exercises more effectively. Don't take light, shallow breaths; always breathe deeply, slowly and rhythmically. You should breathe out (exhale) during effort or when contracting your muscles; and breathe in (inhale) during recovery or when expanding your muscles. Good breathing is the key to developing a high level of aerobic fitness.

Clothing and equipment

Your exercise clothing should be loose and comfortable – not restrictive and tightly fitting. It is best to choose natural fabrics like cotton which allow your skin to 'breathe'

You don't have to buy an expensive tracksuit, leotard or exercise-wear. You can work out, cycle or jog in some shorts or leggings and a baggy T-shirt, although having the right gear might help to motivate you. An exercise bra is very helpful as it provides maximum support and comfort.

The one item that you *must* buy is a good pair of shoes. These may be aerobic, cross-training or running shoes,

depending on the exercise you have chosen. There should be sufficient room for your toes to move inside.

How long will it take?

Don't expect to see results overnight. It will take some time before you see a difference in your body shape, but if you exercise regularly it will happen. You can't expect to get fit quickly after years of neglect.

Set yourself a realistic goal and plan out an exercise programme that will work for you and takes into account what you enjoy doing, how much time you have spare, and your general state of health. Follow our safety guidelines and go for it! Don't be disheartened if it takes longer than you expected. Like lots of other new exercisers, you will soon start to feel good and experience a new sense of well-being.

Warm up first

Never be tempted to start exercising without warming up first. This will gently stretch and warm up your muscles, loosen your joints and increase your flexibility. Stretching out the major muscles will help avoid muscle injury.

Develop a warm-up routine that lasts at least 10 minutes. Incorporate a few aerobic exercises to prepare your heart for strenuous activity. Your heart is a muscle too and it needs to be warmed up.

Cardiovascular exercise

Scientific research shows that cardiovascular exercise strengthens your heart muscle and helps to reduce the risk of heart disease. It also improves circulation and lowers blood pressure.

Strenuous, rhythmic aerobic activity can help prevent a heart attack by making your heart beat faster and harder so that it becomes stronger. A strong heart does not have to work so hard; it can draw oxygen from the blood more efficiently and pump more blood with each beat.

Running, cycling, swimming, rowing, dancing or working out strenuously are all good forms of cardiovascular exercise and will help strengthen your heart. To measure how effectively you are exercising, you can take your pulse rate. This will tell you how your body is responding to exercise. Most of us have a resting pulse rate of 60 to 80 beats a minute, but this increases when we exercise.

Measuring your pulse rate

You can take your pulse rate by pressing a finger to your wrist on the thumb side before you start exercising, during exercise and afterwards. An easy way is to count for 15 seconds and then multiply by four to get the rate per minute. Your pulse rate when you exercise should fall somewhere between your personal maximum and minimum levels.

To work out your maximum level: subtract your age from 200.

To work out your minimum level: subtract your age from 170.

Therefore if you are 40 years old, your training pulse rate should fall in the 130-160 region. If it is less than 130, you are not exercising hard enough; if it exceeds 160, you are training too hard and you should ease up a little.

Improve your posture

Exercise will help improve your posture and prevent muscle pain in the back and joints. Good posture will make you feel better *and* also look slimmer. Instantly you will look as though you have lost several pounds if you stand correctly and walk tall.

It is vital to maintain good posture throughout your exercise programme. To check and correct your posture, stand side on to a full-length mirror.

1 Stand up with feet hip-distance apart.
2 Pull your shoulders back and down, taking a deep breath.
3 Drop your tail bone down.
4 Pull your stomach muscles in.
5 Keep your chest lifted and lengthen spine upwards, increasing the distance between lower rib cage and hip bones.
6 Raise your chin and tuck it in.
7 Check that your pelvis hasn't pushed forwards. Imagine a vertical line passing through head, shoulders, hips and knees.
8 Now breathe in slowly three times on a count of six, hold for six and breathe out for six. Check that your chin is up, your shoulders dropped comfortably.

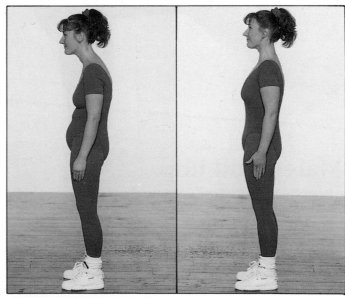

You can make yourself look slimmer by changing your posture. Left: bad posture. Right: good posture.

Warm up

Start your home work-out session with a warm up to get you ready for some action. These warm-up exercises are important as they will prepare your body and stretch out tense muscles, thereby helping to prevent injuries. Even if you don't follow the whole plan every day, it is still a good idea to go through your warm up routine and stretch your muscles.

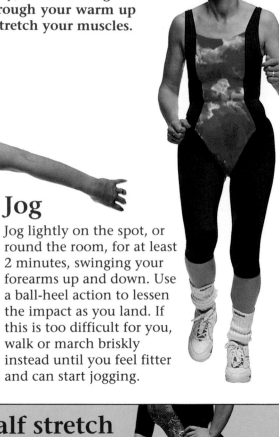

Jog

Jog lightly on the spot, or round the room, for at least 2 minutes, swinging your forearms up and down. Use a ball-heel action to lessen the impact as you land. If this is too difficult for you, walk or march briskly instead until you feel fitter and can start jogging.

Calf stretch

Stand as shown with your feet flat, facing forwards, and the front knee in line with the ankle. Place one hand on your thigh for support and hold for 10 seconds. Repeat with the other leg.

March and hop

March on the spot for 1 minute, raising your knees to hip level and swinging your arms back and forth to shoulder level. If you feel unsteady, try keeping the arms and legs a little lower. As you get fitter, try to extend the movement by introducing a hop.

Squat pumps

Stand with legs hip distance apart and knees and arms bent. Lean on one leg and reach up with the opposite arm and hand. Feel the stretch in your muscles down the side of your body and hold the stretch. Lower your arm and shift to the other leg. Repeat to the other side and alternate pumping left and right for at least 1 minute. This will warm up your thigh muscles.

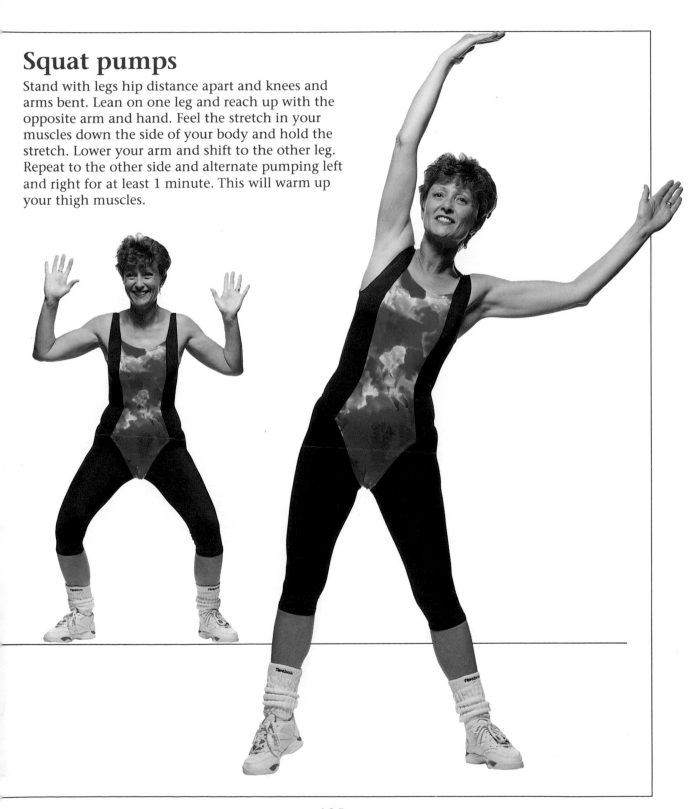

Warm up

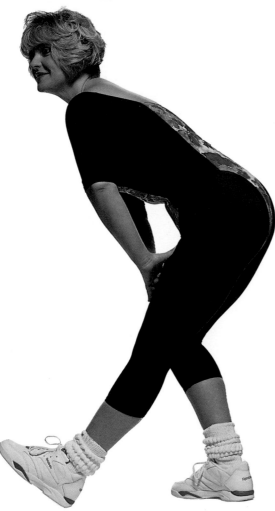

Side stretches

Stand tall with your feet slightly wider than shoulder width apart, your left hand on your thigh. Reach upwards with the right hand, lifting the ribs high. Reach over slightly with the extended arm. Hold for 6-8 seconds and repeat on the other side.

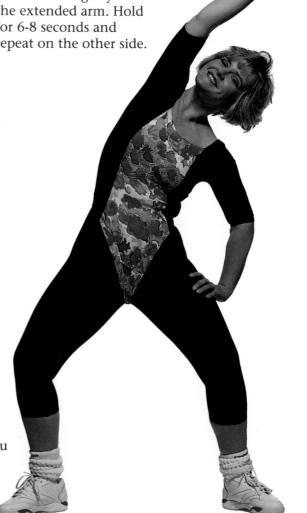

Standing hamstring stretch

Stand facing a wall or door. Bend one knee slightly and extend the other leg in front of you with the toes flexed. Place your hands on the wall or your thighs to support your body weight. Hold the stretch for 8-10 seconds and then change legs and repeat to the other side. Don't lock your front knee; keep your stomach muscles tight.

Upper body ... Chest

The following exercises will tone and strengthen your upper body. They will help firm up slack muscles and improve your upper body shape. Build them into your work-out routine.

Chest presses

With elbows bent, raise your upper arms to shoulder level. Press the arms together and hold for a few seconds. Then spread them again. Repeat 8 times.

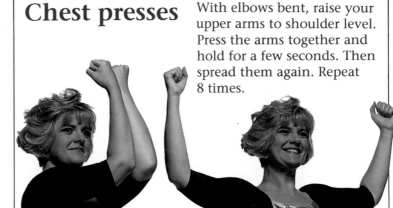

Press ups

Kneel on all fours, hands wide apart and fingers pointing straight ahead. Lean forwards slightly, holding your stomach in, and bend your arms as you lower your face towards the floor. Hold for a few seconds and return to the starting position. You may find this tough, so gradually build up the number of repetitions. Keep your back straight and bottom down; let your arms do the work.

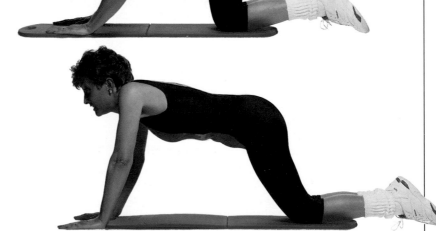

Upper body
... Arms and shoulders

The exercises shown here will firm up your upper arms and shoulders. Many people who have been overweight tend to have problems with their upper arms, and these simple routines are ideal for toning these problem areas. You can buy small weights or improvise with cans.

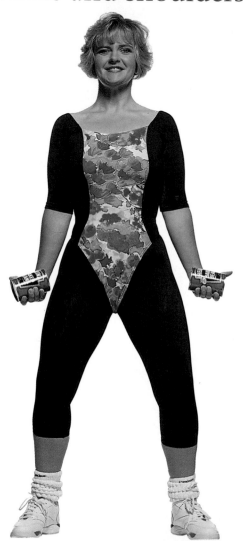

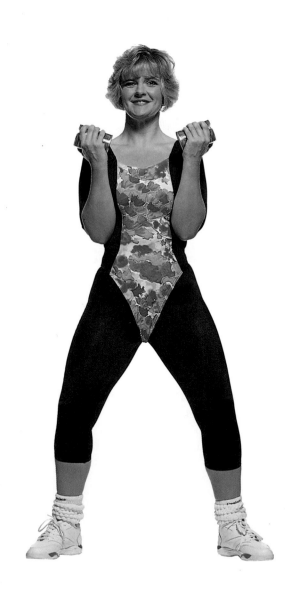

Bicep curls

Stand with your legs apart and knees slightly bent, holding a weight in each hand with palms upward. Keeping your elbows by your sides, bend them and raise your hands to shoulder height. Keep the movement slow and controlled. Repeat 10-12 times.

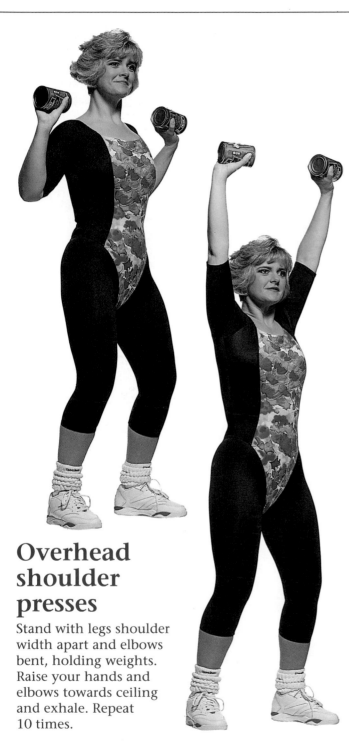

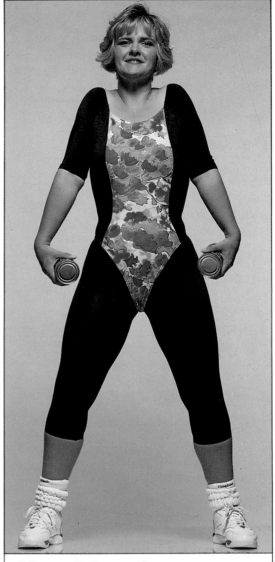

Overhead shoulder presses

Stand with legs shoulder width apart and elbows bent, holding weights. Raise your hands and elbows towards ceiling and exhale. Repeat 10 times.

Shoulder shrugs

Stand with feet hip distance apart, arms by your sides, holding weights and palms facing inwards. Bring your shoulders up towards your ears slowly, keeping your arms straight. Lower your shoulders, and repeat the exercise 10 times. Exhale as you raise your shoulders; inhale as you lower them.

Legs

This set of exercises will work your leg muscles and help tone problem hips and thighs, which might be on the heavy side. They are simple to perform and you will soon see the benefits if you practise them regularly.

Heel raises

Using a chair or table for balance, raise one foot, bending the knee, and lift as high as possible. Rise up on your toes, keeping your back straight and stomach pulled in. Hold for a count of 2 and return to the starting position. Do 8 repetitions each side.

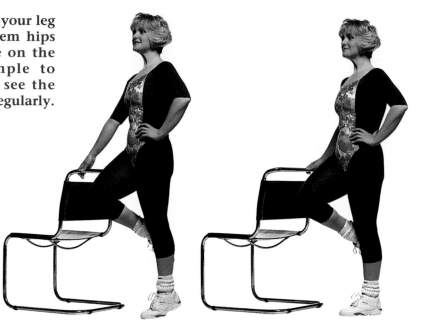

Thigh scoops

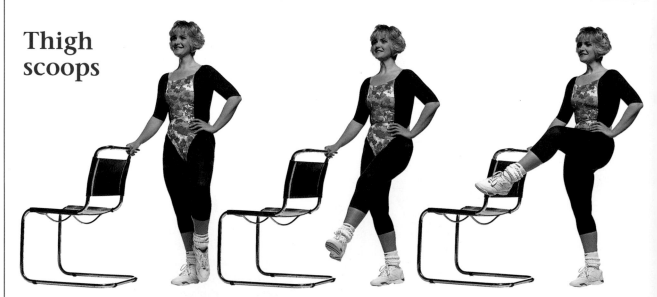

Stand sideways on to a chair, your supporting leg straight and the opposite knee and foot pointing slightly outwards. Swing your leg up and out and then bend the knee and raise it higher and across the supporting leg. Return to the starting position and repeat 8 times. Repeat the sequence with the other leg. This strengthens the front of the thighs and hips.

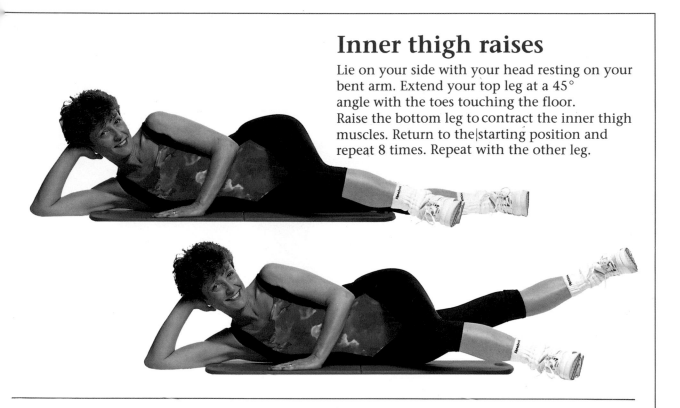

Inner thigh raises

Lie on your side with your head resting on your bent arm. Extend your top leg at a 45° angle with the toes touching the floor. Raise the bottom leg to contract the inner thigh muscles. Return to the starting position and repeat 8 times. Repeat with the other leg.

Outer thigh raises

Lie on your side with the bottom leg slightly bent. Raise and lower the top leg 8 times with toes pointed. Repeat the exercise on the other side.

Buttocks . . .

These exercises will firm up and shape your bottom by toning the muscles in your buttocks. You may find some of them a little difficult at first but as you gradually get fitter, you will be able to stretch further and do more repetitions to work the muscles even harder.

Donkey kicks

Rest on your elbows and knees, stomach pulled in and back flat. Bend the left knee and lift to hip level. Hold for 1 second, lower and repeat 8 times each side. Do not arch your back or lift your leg too high.

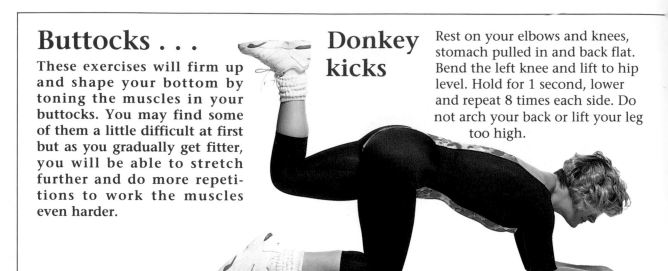

Extended leg lifts

Rest on your elbows and knees, stomach pulled in and back flat. Extend one leg out straight until it is in line with your spine. Do not lift it high; keep the movement smooth and controlled. Repeat 8 times each side.

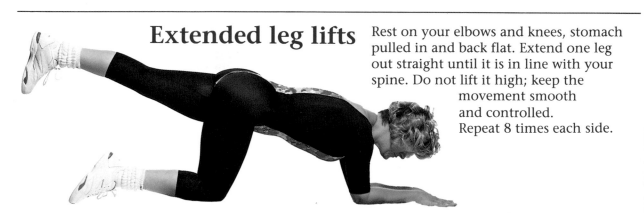

Hip raises

Lie on your back with knees bent and feet hip distance apart. Pull your stomach in and press the small of your back into the floor, squeezing the buttocks together. Now raise them slightly off the floor, still squeezing. Repeat the exercise 8-10 times.

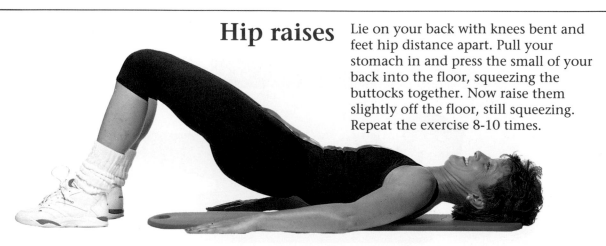

Side raises

Lie on one side, supporting your head on your lower arm, with your legs bent at a 90° angle. Holding your stomach in, raise the top leg without leaning back. Lower and squeeze the thighs together. Repeat 8-10 times and then repeat on the other side.

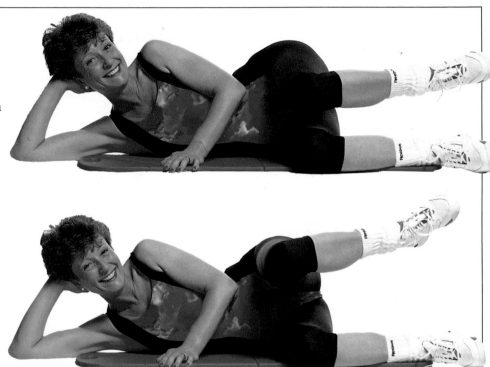

... and stomach

The exercise below and those overleaf will work your abdominal (stomach) muscles. For most of us, this is a very difficult area to firm up, even if you have already lost a lot of weight.

Abdominal curls

Lie flat on your back with your knees bent, feet hip distance apart. Place your hands on the sides of your head and lift the head and shoulders off the floor; do not pull on your neck. Lower and repeat 8-12 times. Move slowly and smoothly, not jerkily.

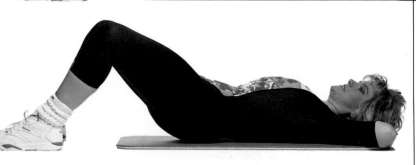

Stomach

Abdominal crunches

Lie on your back, knees bent and feet crossed, with your hands at the sides of your head. Keeping your chin off your chest, gently raise your upper body off the floor, and lower again. Exhale as you lift and inhale as you return. Repeat 10 times.

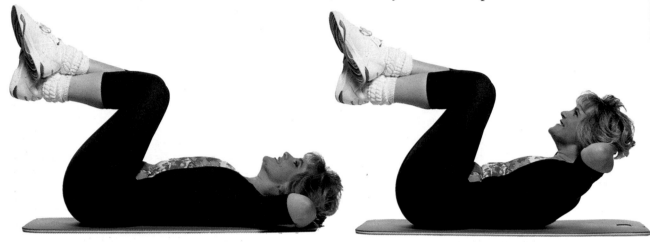

Pelvic tilts

Lie on your back with knees bent and feet flat on the floor. Relax your arms at your sides. Raise your hips towards the ceiling by contracting your lower abdominal muscles. Do not arch your back; the middle of your back should still be on the floor. Slowly lower your bottom to the starting position and repeat 10 times.

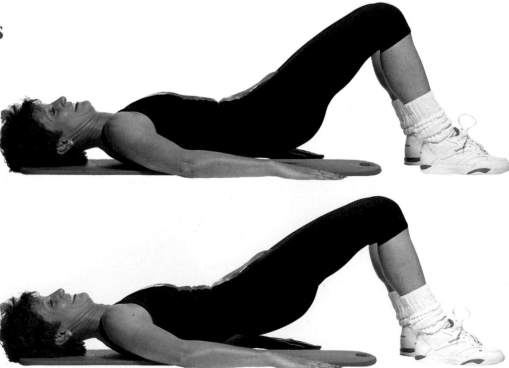

Oblique curl-ups

Adopt the same position, placing both hands behind your head. Pull in your stomach and curl your left shoulder off the floor. Lower yourself to the starting position and repeat 8 times. Then repeat 8 times on the right side. This exercise is good for the waist and stomach.

Abdominal chair curls

Support your lower legs on a chair and slide your bottom in towards the chair. With your hands supporting your head and your neck relaxed, raise your shoulders off the floor and then lower your body to the starting position. Repeat 8 times.

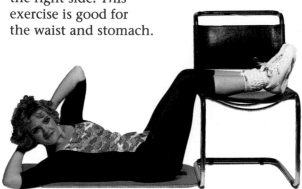

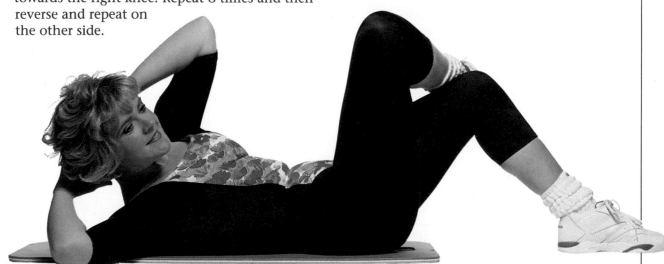

● *Alternative exercise*
Oblique side curls

Alternatively, you can perform the exercise above by crossing your right leg over the left knee and raising the left shoulder off the floor; bring it in towards the right knee. Repeat 8 times and then reverse and repeat on the other side.

Cool down

It is very important to cool down at the end of a work-out and stretch out your muscles. This helps prevent injuries and also relaxes you.

Back of thigh stretch

Lie on your back with one leg bent and foot flat on the floor. Ease the other leg into the chest, keeping the knee as straight as possible. Hold for 20 seconds; repeat on other side. Do 8-10 repetitions.

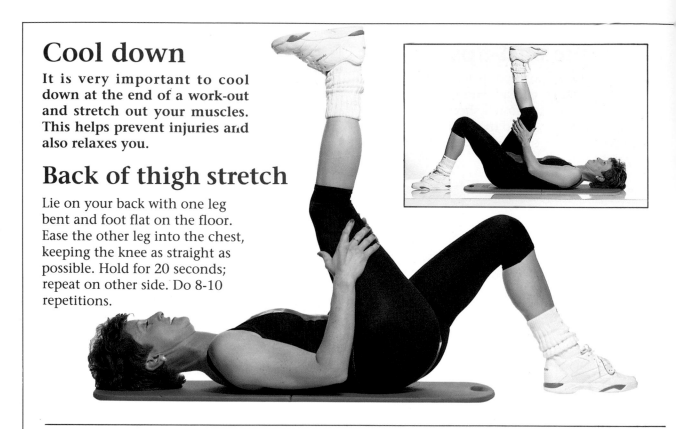

Spine extensions

From a face-down position lying on the floor, lift your upper body, keeping your hips on the floor and supporting your weight on your hands and arms. Hold the stretch for a count of 10 and repeat.

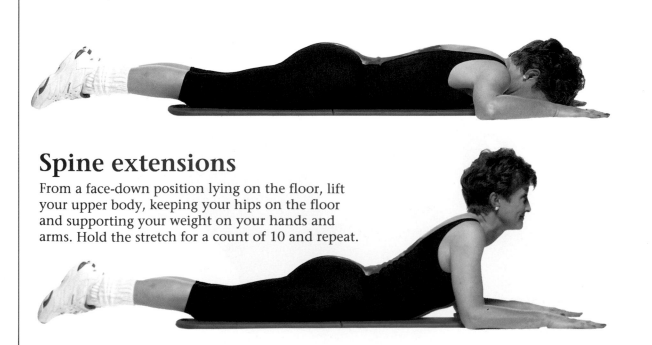

Chest stretches

This can be performed standing (left) or seated. Holding your stomach in tightly, squeeze the shoulder blades back and together without arching your back. Hold for a few seconds and then repeat.

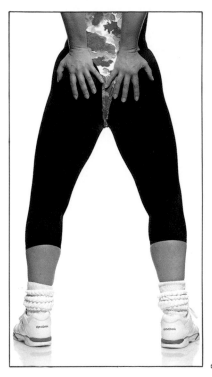

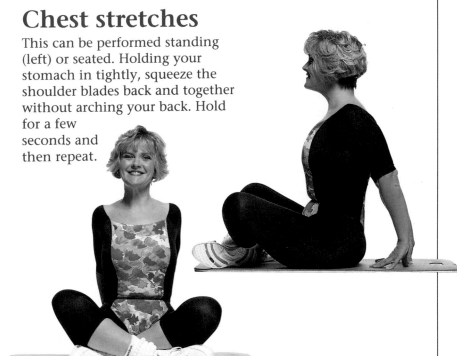

Inner thigh and groin stretch

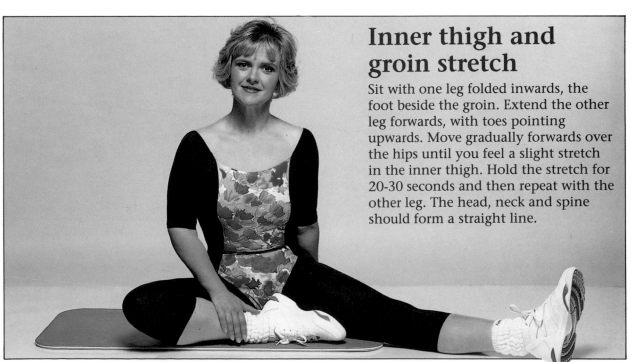

Sit with one leg folded inwards, the foot beside the groin. Extend the other leg forwards, with toes pointing upwards. Move gradually forwards over the hips until you feel a slight stretch in the inner thigh. Hold the stretch for 20-30 seconds and then repeat with the other leg. The head, neck and spine should form a straight line.

On the following pages you will find a complete 14-day Programme which sets out a diet and exercise plan for you to follow. In order to lose weight and be successful, you should do exactly what is recommended. If you try to adapt it or do your own thing, you may not lose weight as rapidly as you would like.

Before you start it is a good idea to weigh yourself and record your starting weight – to do this, follow the guidelines on page 14. Then you can weigh yourself at the end of Week One and again at the end of Week Two. Try not to hop on the scales every day; you will only be disappointed if you cannot see a discernible weight loss from the day before.

Exercise regularly

Regular exercise at least three times a week will help to speed up your weight loss. You can choose whatever you like doing and supplement this with the special exercises that we have included in the Programme. If you have not started exercising yet, maybe doing the

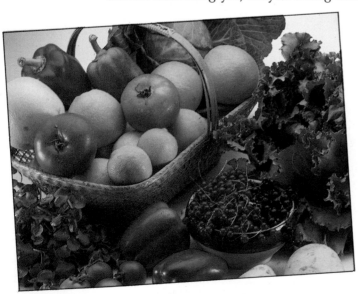

Daily Selections

The Programme is based on eating the following Selections each day:

Women

You should eat 4 Carbohydrate (Bread) Selections, 3 Fat Selections, 3 Fruit Selections, 2 Milk Selections, 5 Protein Selections and 3 Vegetable Selections. (This is the equivalent of approximately 1200 calories per day.)

Men and Young People

Men and young people need extra food. They must add the following every day:

● Add 2oz/60g poultry, meat or oily fish (e.g. salmon or tuna) OR 4oz/120g white fish OR 4oz/120g low-fat soft cheese or smoked or firm tofu OR 6oz/180g beans OR 1oz/30g TVP. You may add these to your lunch or dinner

● Eat one extra piece of fruit, one Fat Selection (see the photo-guide on page 31) and two slices of bread

Note! Young people must add an extra ½ pint/300ml skimmed milk to their daily allowance or 5fl oz/150ml low-fat natural yogurt

exercises in the following pages will inspire you to make exercise a regular part of your weekly routine.

Programme guidelines

● You may use artificial sweetener to sweeten drinks and cereals but no sugar. If you find that the taste of natural yogurt is too sharp, try adding a little sweetener and a few drops of vanilla flavouring to give a creamy taste

● Breakfast cereals may be any type except sugar-coated

Measuring and weighing food

It is essential that you measure all the foods you eat on the plan – do not 'guesstimate' as this will affect your weight loss and may slow it down. When using teaspoons or table-spoons, all spoon measures given must be level.

● You should drink about 6 – 8 glasses of water per day. Half of these can come from tea and coffee. Note: tea or coffee for breakfast is always optional

● Always discard all fat from meat and remove all the skin from poultry

● When using canned or frozen fruit or fruit juices, select only those products that have no added sugar, e.g. canned fruit should be packed in natural juices, not syrup

● When using canned tuna or other fish ensure it is packed in brine, *not* oil

● Various vegetables have been selected but you may choose your own particular favourites from the Vegetables List opposite. However, you must not eat peas, sweetcorn, parsnips, broad beans, sweet potatoes or water chestnuts unless stated in the menu plan

● Meals may be interchanged within the day, or whole days within the week

Eating out

We suggest that you try to avoid eating out if possible while you are following the 14-day Programme, or at least do not do so more than once a week. If you do eat out in a restaurant, eat lightly for the rest of the day and make sensible choices from the menu.

As a starter, you could opt for a small wedge of melon or a small glass of fruit juice (4fl oz/120ml). You could follow this with a small portion of grilled white fish or chicken with vegetables or an undressed salad and a baked potato (but no butter). For a dessert, choose some fresh fruit salad and ice cream.

If you are a vegetarian, you may choose any vegetarian dish but avoid fried foods and creamy sauces.

Vegetarians

We have created a special 14-day menu plan for you to follow. Your daily allowances are exactly the same, and the same diet guidelines apply. Of course, you do not have to be a vegetarian to follow the plan and those people who eat some fish and/or poultry but no red meat can also follow it.

Vegetables

You can eat any of these vegetables with any meal. You can eat them raw, steamed or boiled at any time. Alter-natively, you can substitute them for those suggested on the menu plan.

Artichoke hearts	Mushrooms
Asparagus	Mustard and
Aubergines	cress
Beans, green	Okra
Beansprouts	Onions
Beetroot	Peppers
Broccoli	Pickled vegetables
Brussels sprouts	Pumpkin
Cabbage	Radishes
Carrots	Sauerkraut
Cauliflower	Spinach
Celeriac	Spring onions
Celery	Swede
Chicory	Tomatoes
Courgettes	Tomato juice
Cucumber	(4fl oz/120ml)
Endive	Tomato purée
Fennel	(4 tablespoons)
Leeks	Turnips
Lettuce	Vegetable juice
Mange-tout	(4fl oz/120ml)
Marrow	Watercress

Day 1

Congratulations! Deciding that you really want to lose weight is your first step to success. It is important that you take just one day at a time. You may well be wondering whether or not you will have enough willpower to see this diet through for the whole fourteen days, and there is absolutely no doubt that you can do it if you want to. It may be useful for you later on if today you write down the three most important reasons why you want to lose weight.

BREAKFAST
4fl oz/120ml fruit juice
1oz/30g cereal (not sugar-coated)
¼ pint/150ml skimmed milk

LUNCH
Egg in Tomato Mayonnaise
2oz/60g chunk French bread
4 teaspoons low-fat spread

Dessert: 2½ fl oz/45ml low-fat natural yogurt

DINNER
4oz/120g grilled salmon steak or mackerel
8oz/240g potato
green salad and tomatoes
Dessert: 1 medium apple OR orange OR pear

THROUGHOUT THE DAY
½ pint/300ml skimmed milk

FOOD FOR THOUGHT
You will see that we have incorporated yogurt into many of our suggested meals. Yogurt does not have magical slimming powers but is a good source of calcium and an alternative to milk. If you do not like the low-fat natural variety, try enhancing the flavour with a few drops of vanilla essence and a little artificial sweetener.

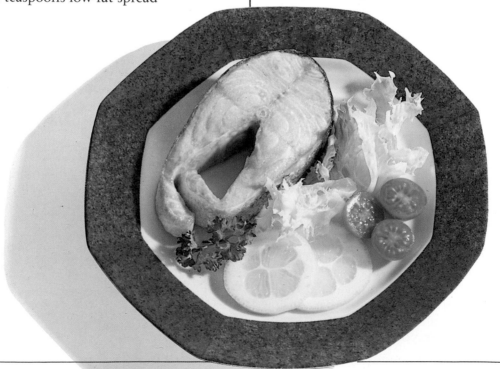

EGG IN TOMATO MAYONNAISE

This is a variation of the usual egg mayonnaise. The addition of tomato ketchup adds both colour and taste. This recipe is ideal as a starter for a main meal but is most useful supplemented with additional crisp lettuce, sliced tomato and cucumber for a filling packed lunch or picnic dish. Who said dieting couldn't be fun!

⅓ teaspoon tomato ketchup
few drops of Worcestershire sauce
1 teaspoon mayonnaise
1 teaspoon low-fat natural yogurt
½ teaspoon single cream
1 small sprig of fresh basil
1 lettuce leaf, shredded
1 egg, hard-boiled, shelled and halved
sprigs of basil to garnish

1   With a fork, mix together the tomato ketchup, Worcestershire sauce, mayonnaise, yogurt and cream. Finely chop the basil and stir into the mayonnaise mixture.
2   Arrange the lettuce on a small serving plate and place the egg halves on top. Spoon a little of the tomato mayonnaise over each half-egg, garnish with sprigs of basil and serve.

Preparation: 10 minutes
Serves 1 *115 calories*
Selections: 1 Fat, 1 Protein, ¼ Vegetable, 15 Optional Calories

Neck mobilizers

Stand with you feet hip distance apart, your knees relaxed and arms by your sides, facing forwards. Relax your shoulders downwards and turn your head to one side. Hold for a second and then turn your head to the other side. Repeat 8 times on each side. This exercise helps loosen your neck muscles and releases tension in this area.

Vegetarian Menu Plan

BREAKFAST
5oz/150g melon
1oz/30g cereal (not sugar-coated)
¼ pint/150ml skimmed milk

LUNCH
1oz/30g slice toast
6oz/180g baked beans
grilled tomato and mushrooms
Dessert: 2½fl oz/75ml low-fat natural yogurt

DINNER
2oz/60g grilled vegetarian sausage
sliced onion, cooked in
1 teaspoon oil
8oz/240g potato
4oz/120g peas
cauliflower, carrots
2fl oz/60ml gravy
Dessert: 4oz/120g peaches

THROUGHOUT THE DAY
½ pint/300ml skimmed milk

Day 2

With Day 1 behind you, Day 2 will seem easier. It is sometimes hard to stop thinking about the food that you enjoy or miss! Today you should think about a short-term goal that you would like to achieve as you shed those unwanted pounds and also decide upon a non-edible reward that would recognise your achievement. Perhaps a new hair style would give you a boost as your face becomes slimmer. Perhaps a manicure would make you feel pampered, or maybe you should delve into your wardrobe to retrieve that favourite outfit in a once comfortable size to convince you that this is the best decision that you have made for a very long time.

BREAKFAST
5oz/150g melon OR 4fl oz/120ml orange juice
1oz/30g slice toast
2 teaspoons low-fat spread
2 teaspoons marmalade

LUNCH
3oz/90g baked beans
1oz/30g slice toast
2 teaspoons low-fat spread
mixed salad
Dessert: 5fl oz/150ml low-fat fruit yogurt

DINNER
3oz/90g grilled turkey sausage
8oz/240g potato
2 teaspoons low-fat spread
onion, tomato
4oz/120g peas
Dessert: 1 medium apple OR orange OR pear

THROUGHOUT THE DAY
½ pint/300ml skimmed milk

FOOD FOR THOUGHT
Skimmed milk is an essential part of any successful diet. It is almost fat-free with approximately half the calories of full-fat milk and your palate will soon adapt to the less creamy taste. Drinking skimmed milk will become a way of life.

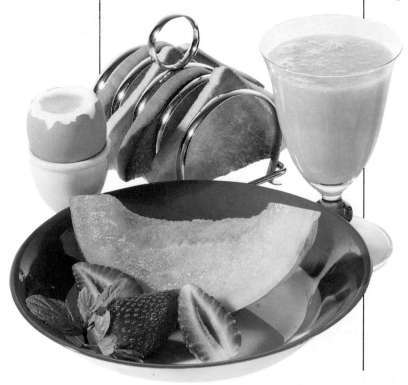

Shoulder circles

Stand with your feet hip distance apart. Make big circles with your arms, swinging them backwards and then forwards. Repeat 8 times, and then perform the exercise again, crossing your hands in front of you as your arms come forwards over your head. This exercise helps to loosen up your shoulders and arms.

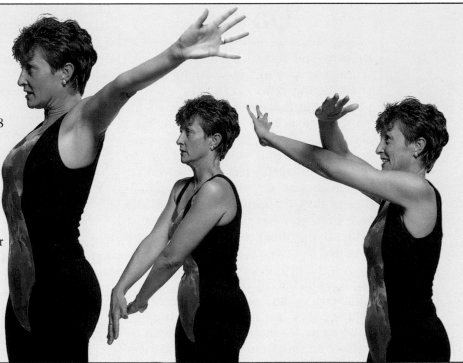

Vegetarian Menu Plan

BREAKFAST
½ medium grapefruit
1oz/30g slice toast
1 tablespoon peanut butter

LUNCH
4fl oz/120ml tomato juice
crispbread up to 120 calories
3 teaspoons low-fat spread
3oz/90g low-fat soft cheese
pickled vegetables
Dessert: 7½ tablespoons low-fat natural yogurt

DINNER
Spinach and Potato Gratin (1 serving)
mixed salad
Dessert: 1 medium peach

THROUGHOUT THE DAY
½ pint/300ml skimmed milk

SPINACH AND POTATO GRATIN

1½lb/720g potatoes, peeled and sliced
salt
1½lb/720g fresh spinach, well-washed
2 teaspoons olive oil
pepper
8oz/240g mature cheese, grated
12oz/360g tomatoes, sliced
2 eggs
5fl oz/150ml low-fat natural yogurt

1 Preheat the oven to 180°C/350°F/Gas Mark 4.
2 Cook the potatoes in boiling, salted water for 5 minutes.
3 Pack the spinach into a large pan with a little salted water. Cover and cook for 4-5 minutes.
4 Drain the spinach really well, squeezing out any excess liquid.
5 Use the olive oil to grease a large shallow ovenproof dish. Layer half the potatoes over the base and season well. Sprinkle with half of the cheese and cover with the spinach. Top with the remaining potatoes, and a layer of sliced tomatoes.
6 Scatter with the rest of the cheese. Beat together the eggs, yogurt and seasoning. Pour over the cheese, and bake for 40-50 minutes.

Preparation: 15 minutes
Cooking: 45-55 minutes
Serves 4 *510 calories per serving*
Selections per serving:
1½ Carbohydrate (Bread), ½ Fat, ¼ Milk, 2½ Protein, 3 Vegetable

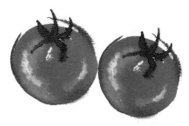

Day 3

By now you should have made a conscious effort to include exercise within your dieting action plan. The exercise programme that we have planned for you on page 96 is effective, fun and, above all, *safe*. Now the fat stores in your body are depleting, you should begin to feel more energetic. It is well known that Day 3 is the day that 'professional' dieters find the most challenging. The fact that you have crossed this most difficult threshold means that you are destined to succeed!

FOOD FOR THOUGHT
Chicken is an excellent source of protein; it is low in fat and extremely good value for money. It is essential to remove all skin from chicken before it is eaten, as 90 per cent of its fat content is found in the skin.

BREAKFAST
4fl oz/120ml orange juice
1 poached egg
1oz/30g slice toast
2 teaspoons low-fat spread

LUNCH
3oz/90g tuna, mashed with
1 teaspoon seafood sauce
crispbreads up to 40 calories
1 teaspoon low-fat spread
celery and watercress
½ medium apple sliced
1½ oz/45g grapes

DINNER
Stir-fried Chicken in Sherry Sauce
6oz/180g cooked pasta or noodles
Dessert: 5fl oz/150ml low-fat natural yogurt

THROUGHOUT THE DAY
½ pint/300ml skimmed milk

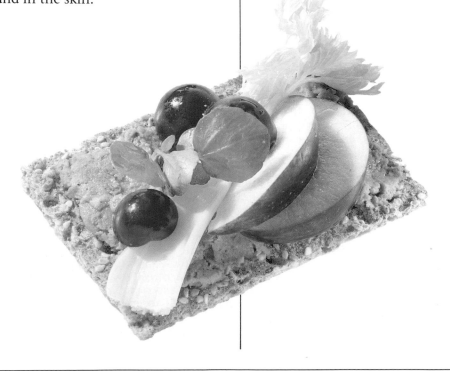

STIR-FRIED CHICKEN IN SHERRY SAUCE

½ tablespoon oil
¼ small onion, finely chopped
1 small clove garlic, finely chopped
3½ oz/105g boned skinned chicken, cut into thin strips
1 tablespoon flour
1½ tablespoons sherry
4fl oz/120ml chicken stock
¼ teaspoon dried tarragon
1½ oz/45g baby button mushrooms, halved
¼ red pepper, deseeded and cut into thin strips
1½ oz/45g drained, canned sweet-corn kernels
salt and pepper

1 Heat the oil in a small saucepan or wok and stir-fry the onion and garlic for 2-3 minutes. Add the chicken and stir-fry for 1-2 minutes.
2 Sprinkle the flour into the saucepan, and gradually blend in the sherry and stock. Add the tarragon, mushrooms, red pepper and sweetcorn. Bring to the boil, stirring well, then cover the saucepan and cook over a low heat for 20 minutes, stirring occasionally to prevent sticking. Season to taste.

Preparation: 5 minutes

Cooking: 30 minutes

Serves 1 *290 calories*

Selections: ½ Carbohydrate (Bread), 1½ Fat, 2½ Protein, 1½ Vegetable, 50 Optional Calories

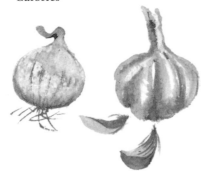

Shoulder presses

Perform this exercise with a broom handle or long stick. Stand with your feet shoulder distance apart, knees slightly bent. Hold the broom handle in both hands behind your shoulders, palms facing forwards, elbows bent. Raise and lower the broom handle slowly behind your shoulders and head. Repeat the exercise 8 times.

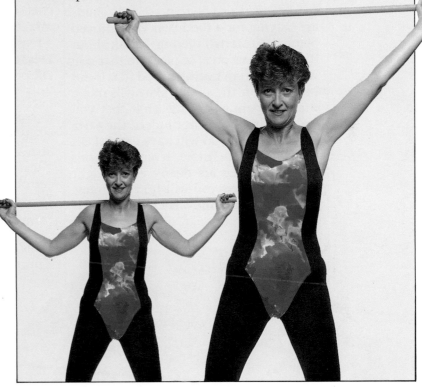

Vegetarian Menu Plan

BREAKFAST
5oz/150g melon
1 boiled egg
1oz/30g slice bread, with
2 teaspoons low-fat spread

LUNCH
1oz/30g pitta bread, filled with
1oz/30g grated cheese
lettuce, tomato, cucumber
2 teaspoons low-calorie mayonnaise

Dessert: 6oz/180g grapes

DINNER
8oz/240g baked jacket potato
2 teaspoons low-fat spread
6oz/180g baked beans
mushroom, tomato, green pepper
Dessert: 5fl oz/150ml low-fat fruit yogurt.

THROUGHOUT THE DAY
½ pint/300ml skimmed milk

Day 4

Over halfway through the first week and by now you should be feeling in control of your eating pattern. You will probably be feeling less tired, and pleased that at long last you are less dependent on food. It may also be that your tastebuds are craving for a food that you enjoyed before you started dieting. Think about it! The few seconds of pleasure that you will enjoy from tasting a food that is not included on the menu plan will in no way compensate for the guilt that you will feel afterwards nor indeed the extra calories which you will have eaten. Plan to enjoy those more tempting foods only when you are nearer your weight loss goal, when you will find them less of a temptation and they will lose their significance.

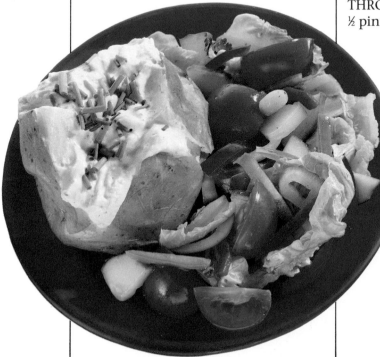

BREAKFAST
½ medium grapefruit
1oz/30g hard cheese, melted on
1oz/30g slice toast

LUNCH
8oz/240g baked jacket potato
2oz/60g cottage cheese OR low-fat soft cheese, sprinkled with chopped chives
mixed salad
4 teaspoons low-calorie mayonnaise
Dessert: 1 medium apple OR orange OR pear

DINNER
3oz/90g grilled pork OR lamb chop OR steak
8oz/240g potato
2 teaspoons low-fat spread
carrots, cabbage
Dessert: 5fl oz/150ml low-fat natural yogurt

THROUGHOUT THE DAY
½ pint/300ml skimmed milk

FOOD FOR THOUGHT
Jacket potatoes are a firm family favourite that can also be enjoyed while losing weight. Contrary to popular belief, potatoes are not fattening; it is the fillings and garnishes that contain the hidden calories. To add taste to your humble baked potatoes substitute low-fat spread for butter, and a combination of low-fat yogurt and herbs for full-fat cream dressings.

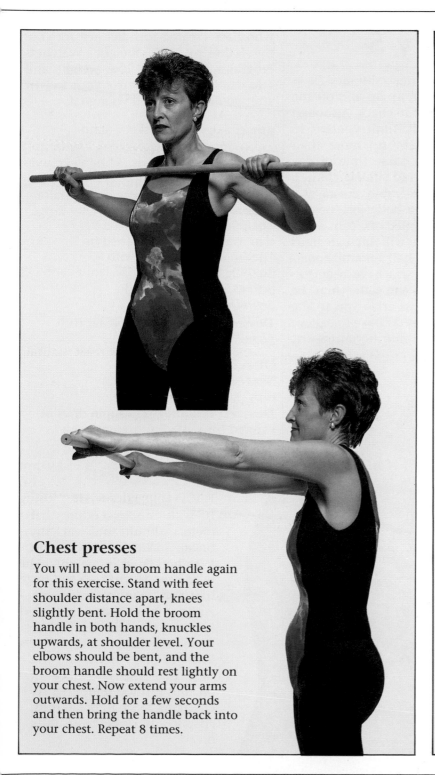

Vegetarian Menu Plan

BREAKFAST
½ medium grapefruit
1oz/30g cereal (not sugar-coated)
¼ pint/150ml skimmed milk

LUNCH
3oz/90g cooked rice, mixed with
6oz/180g canned red kidney beans,
½oz/15g peanuts,
chopped mushrooms and onions
Dessert: 1 medium pear

DINNER
1oz/30g grilled vegetarian burger
3oz/90g baked beans
8oz/240g potato, topped with
1 teaspoon low-fat spread
green beans, onion, tomato
2 teaspoons tomato ketchup
Dessert: 2½fl oz/75ml low-fat natural yogurt

THROUGHOUT THE DAY
½ pint/300ml skimmed milk

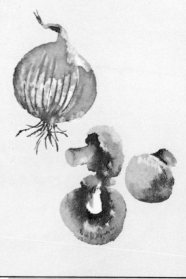

Chest presses

You will need a broom handle again for this exercise. Stand with feet shoulder distance apart, knees slightly bent. Hold the broom handle in both hands, knuckles upwards, at shoulder level. Your elbows should be bent, and the broom handle should rest lightly on your chest. Now extend your arms outwards. Hold for a few seconds and then bring the handle back into your chest. Repeat 8 times.

Day 5

Today you should feel slimmer! It is often tempting to jump on and off the bathroom scales just to check. Although at first it is difficult, limit yourself to checking your weight no more than once a week at the same time of day when you are wearing similar clothes. Weight loss is more rapid during the first few days as the body loses excess fluid before fat is burned off. You can be sure that your weight will fluctuate hour by hour and an odd half a pound apparently gained when you have been following the diet to the letter may be depressing enough to drive you to the biscuit tin! You really do have to believe in yourself and the nutritional experts who have created this diet just for you. By following the Weight Watchers Programme you will lose weight and you will be able to control your weight after you have reached your goal.

BREAKFAST
4fl oz/120ml fruit juice
1oz/30g slice toast
1 tablespoon peanut butter

LUNCH
2oz/60g mushrooms, sliced
½ onion, chopped, stir-fried in
1 teaspoon oil, mixed with
3oz/90g cooked pasta
½oz/15g mashed avocado
2oz/60g ham
Dessert: 5fl oz/150ml low-fat fruit yogurt

DINNER
Seafood Curry (1 serving)
6oz/180g cooked rice
Dessert: 6oz/180g pineapple rings or canned fruit salad in natural juice

THROUGHOUT THE DAY
½ pint/300ml skimmed milk

FOOD FOR THOUGHT
It is a misconception that dieters should not eat any bread. With the Weight Watchers Programme no food is banned since it is essential that you learn to eat in moderation those foods that are higher in calories while increasing your intake of the lower-calorie foods. If you find that the odd slice of bread is just too tempting, try changing to small bread rolls, crispbreads, or delicious pitta bread.

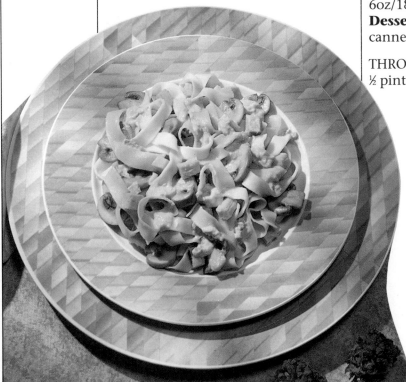

SEAFOOD CURRY

Curries are always a firm family favourite and this one will be no exception. You can replace the fish with chicken if you prefer and, as always, freeze 3 portions for later use if you are eating alone.

1 tablespoon margarine
1 garlic clove, chopped
1 chilli, deseeded and finely chopped
1 teaspoon finely chopped ginger
½ teaspoon ground cumin
½ teaspoon ground coriander
½ teaspoon turmeric
2 medium onions, chopped
8oz/227g canned chopped tomatoes
6fl oz/180ml vegetable stock
1 medium cooking apple
1oz/30g sultanas
10oz/300g skinned white fish, e.g. haddock, monkfish or red mullet fillet
4oz/120g prawns

1 Melt the margarine in a saucepan, add the garlic and stir-fry for 1-2 minutes. Add the chilli (use less chilli if you prefer a mild curry), ginger and spices.
2 Stir the onions, tomatoes and stock into the saucepan.
3 Peel, quarter, core and chop the apple. Add to the mixture with the sultanas, partially cover and simmer for 25 minutes.
4 Cut the fish fillet across the grain into 1½ inch/3.5cm strips. Add the fish strips to the curry sauce, cover and simmer gently for 6-7 minutes.
5 Add the prawns to the curry and simmer for 4 minutes.

Preparation: 10 minutes
Cooking: 40 minutes
Serves 4 *170 calories per serving*
Selections per serving: ½ Fat, ½ Fruit, 1½ Protein, 1½ Vegetable, 10 Optional Calories

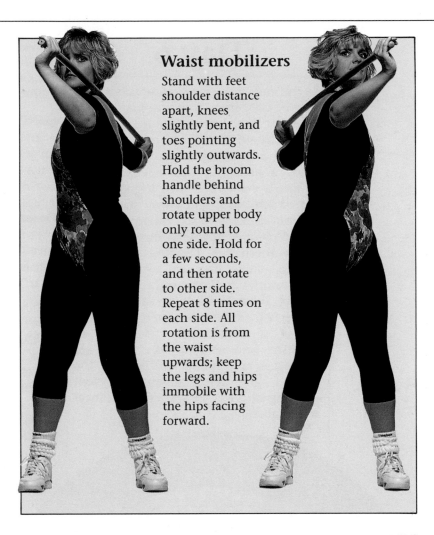

Waist mobilizers

Stand with feet shoulder distance apart, knees slightly bent, and toes pointing slightly outwards. Hold the broom handle behind shoulders and rotate upper body only round to one side. Hold for a few seconds, and then rotate to other side. Repeat 8 times on each side. All rotation is from the waist upwards; keep the legs and hips immobile with the hips facing forward.

Vegetarian Menu Plan

BREAKFAST
5oz/150g melon
1oz/30g cereal (not sugar-coated)
¼ pint/150ml skimmed milk

LUNCH
2oz/60g low-fat soft cheese, spread on
1oz/30g slice bread, with sliced tomato and
2 teaspoons pickle
Dessert: 2½fl oz/75ml low-fat natural yogurt

DINNER
1 small 5 inch/12.5cm corn-on-the-cob
2 teaspoons low-fat spread
6oz/180g cottage cheese mixed salad
2 teaspoons low-calorie mayonnaise
2oz/60g chunk French bread
2 teaspoons low-fat spread
Dessert: 1 medium pear

THROUGHOUT THE DAY
½ pint/300ml skimmed milk

Day 6

As the end of the week approaches, you may be concerned that you may 'break' your diet by accepting that invitation to visit a friend for dinner or to enjoy a meal in a restaurant. If you do wish to enjoy a meal out this week, try and choose a restaurant with a good salad bar or selection, and enjoy your salad without dressing to accompany a lightly grilled piece of fish or poultry or a vegetarian alternative. Puddings should be avoided since they are usually laden with calories and may well weaken your resolve. Fresh fruit is a far safer alternative. If you are accepting an invitation to eat at a friend's, do telephone in advance and explain that you are dieting. A true friend will be only too pleased to help, given sufficient warning, and will see preparing the meal as a challenge.

BREAKFAST
5oz/150g melon
1oz/30g cereal (not sugar-coated)
¼ pint/150ml skimmed milk

LUNCH
3oz/90g tuna
mixed salad
3 teaspoons low-calorie mayonnaise
1oz/30g bap
1 teaspoon low-fat spread
Dessert: 2½ fl oz/75ml low-fat natural yogurt mixed with 1 medium apple, sliced, drizzled with
½ teaspoon honey, scattered with
½ oz/15g toasted almonds

DINNER
3oz/90g grilled lamb OR pork chop OR chicken
8oz/240g potato
broccoli, cabbage
3oz/90g sweetcorn

THROUGHOUT THE DAY
½ pint/300ml skimmed milk

FOOD FOR THOUGHT
Red meats, such as pork, lamb and beef, have a high fat content and for this reason should always be grilled on a rack to allow the excess fat to drip away. Never stir-fry red meats nor roast them with added fat in the oven as this adds unnecessary calories and will raise your fat level intake above the maximum recommended for healthy eating.

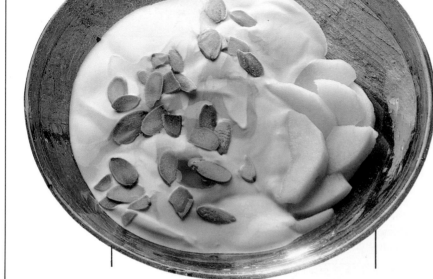

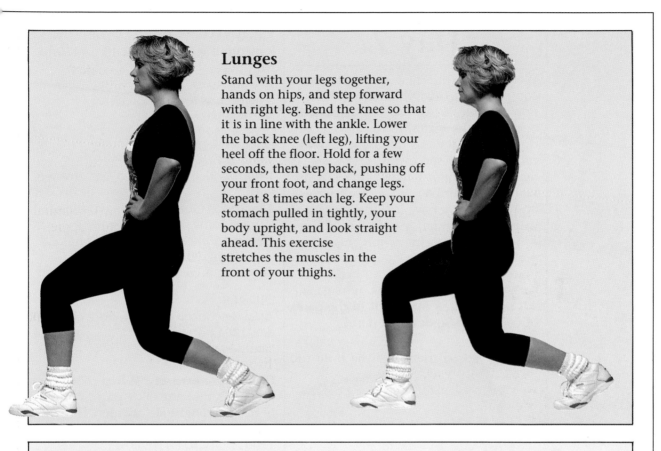

Lunges

Stand with your legs together, hands on hips, and step forward with right leg. Bend the knee so that it is in line with the ankle. Lower the back knee (left leg), lifting your heel off the floor. Hold for a few seconds, then step back, pushing off your front foot, and change legs. Repeat 8 times each leg. Keep your stomach pulled in tightly, your body upright, and look straight ahead. This exercise stretches the muscles in the front of your thighs.

Vegetarian Menu Plan

BREAKFAST
4fl oz/120ml orange juice
1oz/30g slice toast, with
1 teaspoon low-fat spread
mushrooms, cooked in
1 teaspoon oil

LUNCH
Houmous and Pitta Bread
(1 serving)
whole baby tomatoes,
carrot sticks
Dessert: 1 medium apple

DINNER
2-egg cheese and onion
omelette, made with
1oz/30g cheese, cooked in
1 teaspoon oil

8oz/240g potato
4oz/120g peas
broccoli
Dessert: 5fl oz/150ml low-fat
fruit yogurt

THROUGHOUT THE DAY
½ pint/300ml skimmed milk

HOUMOUS AND PITTA BREAD

12oz/360g drained, canned chick peas
2 tablespoons reserved liquid
2 tablespoons lemon juice
1 garlic clove, crushed
2 teaspoons sesame or olive oil
salt and pepper
4 x 1oz/30g pieces of pitta bread

1 Blend the chick peas and the reserved liquid from the can with the lemon juice, garlic and oil in a food processor until smooth.
2 Season to taste, adding extra lemon juice if necessary.
3 Serve with fingers of the warm pitta bread.

Preparation: 5 minutes

Serves 4 *170 calories per serving*

Selections per serving:
1 Carbohydrate (Bread), ½ Fat,
1 Protein

Day 7

Well done! Your first week has been completed successfully and you should now be able to see the results of your efforts on the scales. If you have come this far then there is no doubt that you can be just as successful next week. It really is important that you recognise your success and reward yourself accordingly. Today we have included a glass of wine for you to enjoy with your dinner or lunch but you may omit this if you prefer. This may also be a good day to invest in a new lipstick, a special bubble bath or an interesting book or magazine – if not all three! Success is in the palm of your hand, so don't let it go!

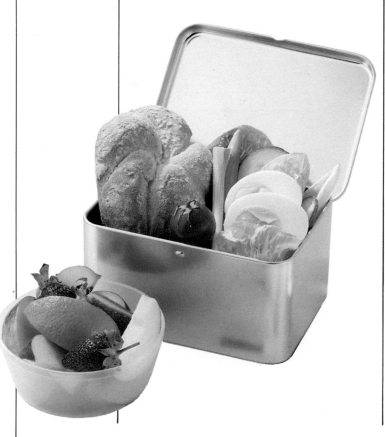

BREAKFAST
½ medium grapefruit OR 4fl oz/120ml fruit juice
1oz/30g toast
2 teaspoons low-fat spread
3oz/90g baked beans

LUNCH
1oz/30g bread roll
1 hard-boiled egg, halved and covered with
4 teaspoons low-calorie mayonnaise
lettuce, tomato, cucumber
Dessert: 5fl oz/150ml low-fat natural yogurt, mixed with
4oz/120g mixed fruit salad

DINNER
3oz/90g cooked chicken
4oz/120g potato
cauliflower, carrots
4oz/120g peas
Chocolate Orange Whip (1 serving)
4fl oz/120ml wine OR ½ pint/300ml beer, bitter, light ale or cider

THROUGHOUT THE DAY
½ pint/300ml skimmed milk

FOOD FOR THOUGHT
Giving up chocolate may seem to be an impossible dieting task to the committed chocoholic. Don't panic! In moderation, chocolate can be enjoyed on the Weight Watchers Programme. It is for this reason that at the end of your first week of dieting, we have included a low-calorie chocolate dessert. If you still crave the pleasurable taste that chocolate brings, try drinking an occasional cup of low-calorie hot chocolate, but remember to count those calories!

CHOCOLATE ORANGE WHIP

Chocoholics will love this sumptuous dessert. If you're eating alone, the freezer will really come into its own. Eat one serving now and freeze 3 servings for delicious desserts in the future.

1 tablespoon cocoa powder
2 tablespoons hot water
1oz/30g plain chocolate, broken into pieces
8oz/240g low-fat soft cheese
grated rind and juice of ½ medium orange
2 egg whites (or 4 teaspoons dried egg white mixed with 2fl oz/60ml water)
2 teaspoons caster sugar
½ medium orange, sliced to decorate

1 In a small bowl, blend the cocoa powder with the hot water, and then add the pieces of chocolate. Place the bowl over a pan of simmering water until the chocolate melts, stirring until smooth. Cool slightly.
2 Beat the soft cheese and then add the orange rind and juice, mixing well. Blend in the chocolate mixture.
3 In a clean bowl, whisk the egg whites until stiff, and then add the caster sugar and whisk again until glossy. Fold in the chocolate mixture thoroughly, using a metal spoon.
4 Divide between 4 serving glasses and chill for 20 minutes. Decorate with orange slices.

Preparation: 15 minutes plus chilling time
Serves 4 *195 calories per serving*
Selections per serving:
1 Protein, 80 Optional Calories

Hip flexes

You will need a chair or table for this exercise for support. Stand side-on to it, with your hand resting on it. Slightly bend the knee of the leg nearer to the chair (or table), and raise your other leg, bending it in towards your body. Flex your raised foot and hold for a few seconds. Lower and repeat 8 times on each side. Make sure that you hold your stomach muscles in tightly throughout this exercise and keep your back relaxed and straight with hips facing forward.

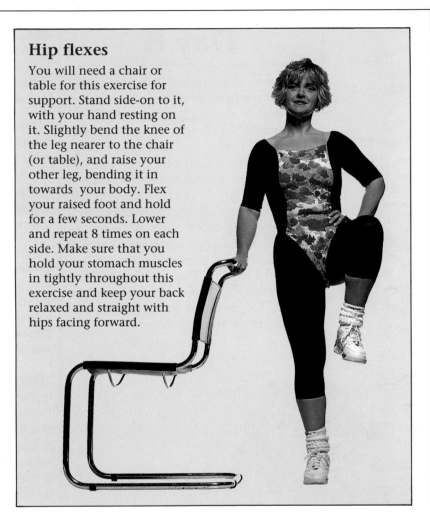

Vegetarian Menu Plan

BREAKFAST
4fl oz/120ml grapefruit juice
1oz/30g cereal (not sugar-coated)
¼ pint/150ml skimmed milk

LUNCH
4oz/120g low-fat soft cheese
2 x 1oz/30g slices bread
tomato, radish, celery
Dessert: 1 medium apple

DINNER
beansprouts, mushrooms, green pepper, stir-fried in 1 teaspoon oil mixed with
1oz/30g cashew nuts
6oz/180g canned kidney beans
6oz/180g cooked rice
2½fl oz/75ml low-fat natural yogurt

THROUGHOUT THE DAY
½ pint/300ml skimmed milk

Day 8

And a new week begins! By now exercise should be part of your routine each day, whether in the form of a set exercise programme or simply by the greater amount of exercise that your body undertakes on a daily basis. Are you still taking the lift or escalator at the office or when you go shopping? Walking up stairs will burn off calories without you even noticing. How often do you take the car for local trips when a walk would be as quick and more effective? When was the last time you used a skipping rope or swam in the local pool? Exercise can be fun, and the more weight you lose the more you will enjoy it.

BREAKFAST
4fl oz/120ml fruit juice
1oz/30g slice toast
2 teaspoons low-fat spread
boiled or grilled mushrooms

LUNCH
1oz/30g slice toast
6oz/180g baked beans
2 x ½oz/15g rashers lean back bacon
2 teaspoons low-fat spread
Dessert: 1 medium apple OR orange OR pear

DINNER
Cheese and Potato Pie
4oz/120g peas
mixed salad
2 teaspoons low-calorie mayonnaise
Dessert: 5fl oz/150ml low-fat natural yogurt

THROUGHOUT THE DAY
½ pint/300ml skimmed milk

FOOD FOR THOUGHT
Breakfast is one of the most important meals of the day and yet unfortunately it is the meal that dieters are most likely to skip. This meal literally breaks the fast since the last meal of the previous evening which could be as long as 12 hours ago. A light breakfast will take only a few minutes to prepare and yet this will stop you feeling hungry mid-morning when temptation may rear its ugly head.

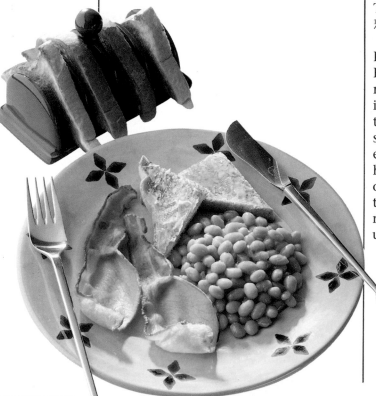

CHEESE AND POTATO PIE

This dish can be enjoyed by all the family. Simply multiply the ingredients by the number you wish to serve.

8oz/240g potatoes
salt
1oz/30g curd cheese
1 tablespoon skimmed milk
a little fresh chervil, finely chopped
few fresh chives, finely chopped
1oz/30g hard cheese, e.g. Cheddar or Double Gloucester, grated
salt and pepper
1 tomato, thinly sliced

1 Cook the potatoes in boiling salted water, then drain well. Mash them with the curd cheese, milk and herbs. Reserve half the hard cheese and mix the remainder into the mashed potatoes. Season with salt and pepper.
2 Spoon the potato mixture into a small flameproof dish and roughen the surface with a fork. Arrange the tomato on top of the potato and sprinkle with the reserved cheese. Cook under a hot grill until golden brown.

Preparation: 10 minutes

Cooking: 20 minutes

Serves 1 *330 calories*

Selections: 2 Carbohydrate (Bread), 1½ Protein, ½ Vegetable, 5 Optional Calories

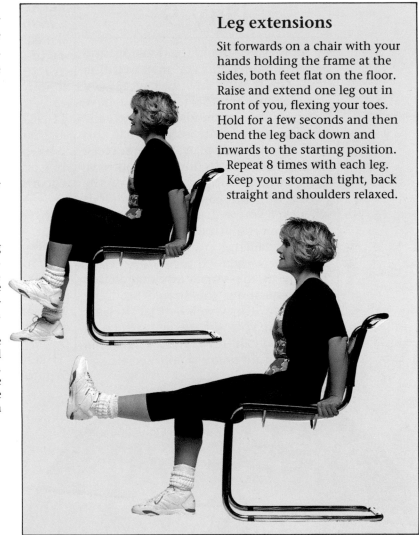

Leg extensions

Sit forwards on a chair with your hands holding the frame at the sides, both feet flat on the floor. Raise and extend one leg out in front of you, flexing your toes. Hold for a few seconds and then bend the leg back down and inwards to the starting position. Repeat 8 times with each leg. Keep your stomach tight, back straight and shoulders relaxed.

Vegetarian Menu Plan

BREAKFAST
4fl oz/120ml grapefruit juice
2 x 1oz/30g slices toast
2 teaspoons low-fat spread
4 teaspoons marmalade

LUNCH
crispbread up to 80 calories

2 tablespoons peanut butter
tomato, cucumber
Dessert: 1 medium pear

DINNER
8oz/240g baked jacket potato
6oz/180g baked beans
tomato, watercress

Dessert: 5fl oz/150ml low-fat natural yogurt

THROUGHOUT THE DAY
½ pint/300ml skimmed milk

Day 9

By now you should be looking and feeling slimmer and you may well find your family and friends paying you compliments. The fact that you have lost only a few pounds is not actually significant; it is the feeling that this gives you that is the key to your success. You will now be feeling that you have the power to succeed. You have the power to refuse any tempting foods whenever you wish and you also have the power to achieve this particular dieting challenge. You should remember this when those non-dieting 'friends' try to persuade you that dieting is not the thing you should be doing right now. It may well be that they are afraid that you will succeed, which of course you will! It won't be long before they will want to know your secret.

BREAKFAST
½ medium banana, sliced
½ medium orange, segmented
1½oz/45g grapes, halved
1oz/30g muesli
¼ pint/150ml skimmed milk

LUNCH
1oz/30g slice bread, spread with
2 teaspoons low-fat spread
pile on top 2oz/60g low-fat soft cheese
cucumber, tomato, onion, pepper rings

DINNER
12oz/360g baked jacket potato
4 teaspoons low-fat spread
1oz/30g grated cheese
3oz/90g grilled turkey or chicken steak
onion, tomato
Dessert: 2½ fl oz/75ml low-fat natural yogurt

THROUGHOUT THE DAY
½ pint/300ml skimmed milk

FOOD FOR THOUGHT
Full-fat hard cheese can be a dieter's downfall. You should have no more than 14oz/420g total of hard cheese and red meat in any one week if you want to lose weight and eat healthily. Cheese, such as cottage or low-fat soft cheese spread, is a pleasant low-calorie alternative which will still satisfy the cheese lover's palate. Try adding herbs, curry powder or interesting flavourings to low-fat soft cheese to stimulate your tastebuds and satisfy your appetite.

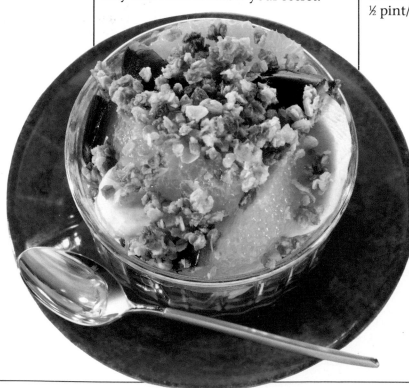

Quad stretches

Lie down flat on your stomach with your head on your hands. Extend your left arm back and grasp your left ankle, bringing your heel into the left buttock. Hold the stretch for 20 seconds. Feel the stretch in the muscles at the front of your thigh. If you can't reach your foot, bring your heel as close to your buttock as you can. Repeat 5 times each side.

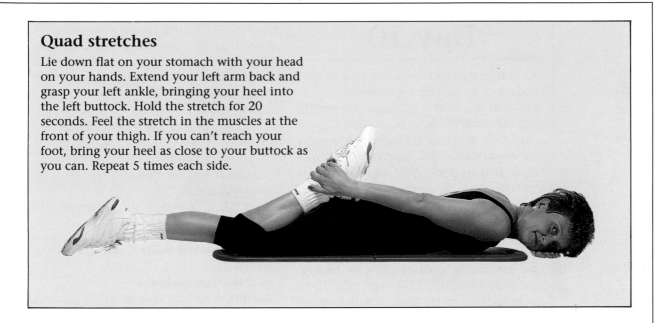

VEGETABLE MOUSSAKA

1 aubergine, sliced
salt
4 teaspoons margarine
1 onion, chopped
1 carrot, chopped
2 celery sticks, sliced
1 medium courgette, sliced
1 red pepper, deseeded and chopped
8oz/240g mushrooms, sliced
14oz/420g canned chopped tomatoes
6oz/180g canned red kidney beans, drained
3fl oz/90ml vegetable stock
freshly ground black pepper
1lb/480g potatoes, cooked and sliced
2 eggs
5fl oz/150ml low-fat natural yogurt
4oz/120g fromage frais (8% fat)

1 Sprinkle the aubergine with salt. Leave for 10-15 minutes, then turn over and repeat. Rinse, drain and pat dry.
2 Preheat the oven to 190°C/375°F/Gas Mark 5.
3 Heat the margarine and stir-fry the onion for 3 minutes. Add the carrot, celery, courgette and red pepper. Cover and cook gently for 5 minutes.
4 Add the mushrooms, tomatoes, kidney beans and vegetable stock. Bring to the boil, then simmer, uncovered for 5 minutes. Season to taste.
5 Pour half of this mixture into an ovenproof casserole and cover with the aubergines. Pour over the remaining mixture and arrange the potatoes on top.
6 Beat the eggs, yogurt and fromage frais. Season and pour over the potatoes. Bake for 45 minutes until set.

Preparation: 20 minutes

Cooking: 1 hour

Serves 4 *250 calories per serving*

Selections per serving:
1 Carbohydrate (Bread), 1 Fat, ¼ Milk, 1½ Protein, 3 Vegetable

Vegetarian Menu Plan

BREAKFAST
3oz/90g banana
1oz/30g cereal (not sugar-coated)
7½ tablespoons low-fat natural yogurt

LUNCH
2oz/60g chunk French bread
4 teaspoons low-fat spread
2½ oz/75g cheese
3 teaspoons pickle
pickled onions, celery, tomato
Dessert: 1 medium apple

DINNER
4fl oz/120ml tomato juice
Vegetable Moussaka
(1 serving)
Dessert: 4oz/120g pineapple

THROUGHOUT THE DAY
½ pint/300ml skimmed milk

Day 10

Do you remember how on Day 1 you made a note of the three most important reasons that you have for losing weight? Today might be a good day to look back at those reasons to give you the inspiration that you need to continue. It is important to remember that not everyone is perfect all the time. There may be occasions when you are losing weight when you slip up and temporarily 'go off the rails'. If at any time you do find yourself slipping and you are losing control of your eating, *just stop*. Consider how well you have done so far, and try and picture in your mind's eye just how you will look and feel when you have lost weight. Get yourself away from any difficult dieting situations and start again from that moment. Learning to regain control is an invaluable experience and one that will help you when you want to maintain your weight loss in the future.

BREAKFAST
½ medium banana OR 4fl oz/120ml fruit juice
1oz/30g slice toast
1 teaspoon low-fat spread
2 teaspoons jam
5fl oz/150ml low-fat natural yogurt

LUNCH
Omelette with Sour Cream and Chives
1oz/30g French bread
1 teaspoon low-fat spread
Dessert: 1 medium apple OR orange OR pear

DINNER
6oz/180g grilled cod or halibut, brushed with 1 teaspoon oil
8oz/240g potato
courgettes, tomatoes, onions

THROUGHOUT THE DAY
½ pint/300ml skimmed milk

FOOD FOR THOUGHT
You will see that today we have suggested a wonderful sour cream and chive omelette for lunch. Herbs are a welcome addition to food at any time, but particularly so to the dieter who is, perhaps, trying new foods and flavours for the first time. With fresh herbs now available in most supermarkets, why not try adding them to soups and casseroles, lightly sprinkled on fish or meat or within a fresh green salad?

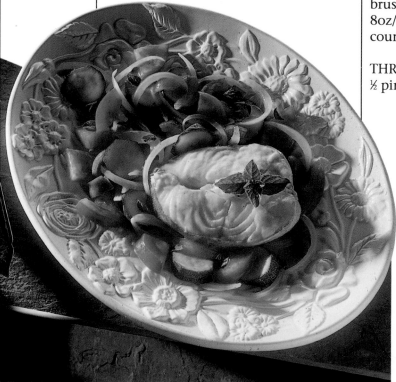

OMELETTE WITH SOUR CREAM AND CHIVES

Omelettes are the dieter's dream; they are quick to prepare and can be transformed with lots of different fillings. If you prefer, you can use 1 egg for this omelette and add 1oz/30g hard cheese or 2oz/60g cottage cheese.

2 eggs
1 teaspoon margarine
1 tablespoon chopped fresh chives
salt and pepper
1 tablespoon sour cream

1 Beat the eggs (with 2 tablespoons of water if wished).
2 Heat the margarine in an omelette pan and pour in the eggs. Scatter half the chives on top, season and cook until set.
3 Mix the remaining chives with the sour cream. Turn out the omelette on to a warmed plate and fold over. Serve with the sour cream and chives.

Preparation: 3 minutes
Cooking: 4-5 minutes
Serves 1 *250 calories*
Selections: 1 Fat, 2 Protein, 50 Optional Calories

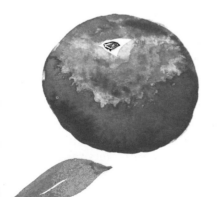

Buttocks stretch and release

This stretch will release the muscles in your buttocks after performing the exercises in the home work-out (see page 112). Sit up straight with your legs extended in front of you. Cross and bend your right leg over extended left leg, with right foot flat on the floor. Support your body with your right arm, and turn head and shoulders to the right with left arm across your body, and left hand resting on right hip. Hold for 20 seconds and repeat on other side.

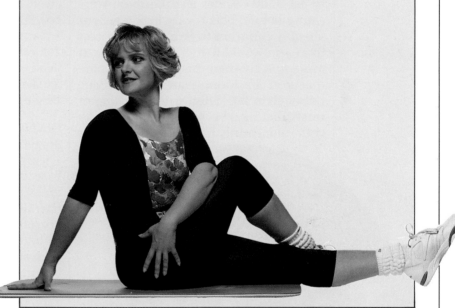

Vegetarian Menu Plan

BREAKFAST
1oz/30g slice toast
2 teaspoons low-fat spread
1 poached egg
grilled mushrooms

LUNCH
2oz/60g low-fat soft cheese
2oz/60g bap
cucumber, onion, tomato
Dessert: 1 medium orange

DINNER
2oz/60g vegetarian sausage
8oz/240g potato
broccoli, carrots
Dessert: 4oz/120g pineapple
5fl oz/150ml low-fat fruit yogurt

THROUGHOUT THE DAY
½ pint/300ml skimmed milk

Day 11

It is a simple fact that if you eat more food and thereby more calories than your body needs, the excess calories will be turned into fat and stored in your body. If you eat fewer calories than your body needs you will lose weight. In order to lose one pound of fat you need to eat 3500 calories less than you were eating before. This is why losing weight sensibly can seem to be a slower process than you would like. If you lose weight more quickly than this, the chances are that you are losing lean muscle tissue rather than fat. Often with this type of crash dieting you soon revert back to your old eating habits. However, this time the lean muscle that you have lost is replaced with fat, and hence the difficulty of dieting a second, third and fourth time around!

BREAKFAST
½ medium banana
1oz/30g cereal (not sugar-coated)
¼ pint/150ml skimmed milk

LUNCH
1oz/30g pitta bread, spread with
1 teaspoon low-fat spread, filled with
2oz/60g corned beef or ham
salad
3 teaspoons low-calorie mayonnaise
Dessert: 1 medium pear

DINNER
3oz/90g cooked chicken, stir-fried in
1 teaspoon oil with
broccoli, red, yellow and green peppers
and spring onions
6oz/180g cooked rice, mixed with
2oz/60g peas
1½ oz/45g sweetcorn kernels
Dessert: 2½ fl oz/75ml low-fat natural yogurt

THROUGHOUT THE DAY
½ pint/300ml skimmed milk

FOOD FOR THOUGHT
Rice and pasta are a filling alternative to bread and potatoes. It is worth remembering that 1oz/30g dried pasta or rice produces 3oz/90g cooked pasta or rice. Left-over cold pasta makes a lovely ingredient with a mixed salad or in a home-made soup. Pasta can now be bought in many interesting shapes and colours in local supermarkets, and the different types of rice, such as basmati or arborio, are worth trying for their taste and different textures.

Inside thigh firmers

Sit up straight on a chair with your hands resting on the frame behind you. Place a cushion between your knees and thighs, and bring your feet and legs together. Looking straight ahead and sitting very erect with stomach muscles pulled in tightly, gently squeeze inwards and release your thigh muscles. Repeat 10 times. This exercise will help to firm up and tone the inner thighs.

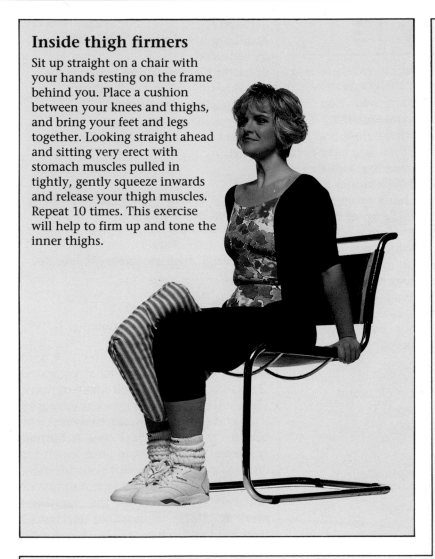

NUTTY SPAGHETTI

4oz/120g spaghetti
salt
2 tablespoons peanut butter
3 tablespoons skimmed milk
1oz/30g roasted peanuts, chopped

1 Cook the spaghetti in boiling salted water until tender.
2 Place the peanut butter in a bowl, and gradually blend in the milk. Add the peanuts.
3 Drain the hot spaghetti, and mix in the peanut mixture thoroughly.

Preparation: 5 minutes

Cooking: 10-15 minutes

Serves 4 *395 calories per serving*

Selections per serving:
2 Carbohydrate (Bread), 2 Fat, 1½ Protein, 10 Optional Calories

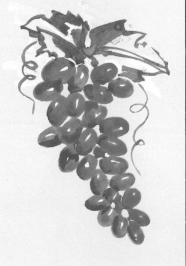

Vegetarian Menu Plan

BREAKFAST
3oz/90g fromage frais
1oz/30g slice toast
2 teaspoons jam

LUNCH
2-egg herb and mushroom omelette, cooked in
1 teaspoon oil
tomato, lettuce

Dessert: 1 medium peach

DINNER
Nutty Spaghetti (1 serving)
4oz/120g peas
side salad
Dessert: 3oz/90g grapes
5fl oz/50ml low-fat natural yogurt

THROUGHOUT THE DAY
½ pint skimmed milk

Day 12

One of the most often heard comments from dieters new to Weight Watchers is 'I've never eaten so much!' You may well be finding that you are eating foods that you have not tried before and that you are eating more than you have done for a long time. The diet that you are following is based on 1200 calories per day for women and a high proportion of those calories are made up of fruit and vegetables which tend to be lower in calories than carbohydrates, such as bread, rice, pasta; or protein, such as cheese, fish and meat. If you do find that you are still hungry when following the meals that we have suggested, you may fill yourself up with vegetables taken from the list on page 119.

BREAKFAST
1 inch/2.5cm wedge melon and
2½ oz/75g strawberries OR
4fl oz/120ml fruit juice
1 boiled egg
1oz/30g slice toast
2 teaspoons low-fat spread

LUNCH
4oz/120g low-fat soft cheese OR tuna mixed salad
2 teaspoons low-calorie mayonnaise
1oz/30g roll (or up to 80 calories crispbreads)
2 teaspoons low-fat spread
Dessert: 5fl oz/150ml low-fat fruit yogurt

DINNER
4 x 1oz/30g breadcrumbed fish fingers
6oz/180g baked beans
6oz/180g potato
tomato, green beans
Dessert: 1 medium apple OR orange OR pear

THROUGHOUT THE DAY
½ pint/300ml skimmed milk

FOOD FOR THOUGHT
Most of the lunches we have suggested are no-cook, no-fuss food combinations. This is to enable you to pack them easily if you take a packed lunch to work, or to prepare them quickly if time is limited at home. You may swap your lunch for dinner on any day to suit your lifestyle. If you eat in the company restaurant or canteen try and match the suggested meal as closely as possible and avoid fried food and cream sauces. If in doubt, ask for a salad.

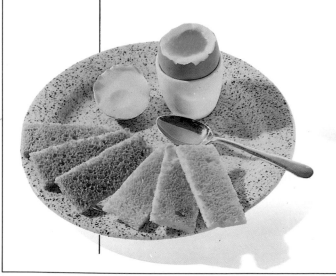

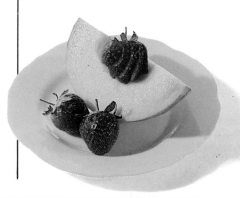

Pectoral stretches

Sit up straight on a chair, knees and feet together, and stomach muscles pulled in tightly. With your arms bent and elbows at shoulder level, hold a cushion or telephone directory between your arms as shown. Gently squeeze and release, feeling the stretch in your upper arms and shoulders. Exhale as you squeeze and bring your elbows together; inhale as you release them.

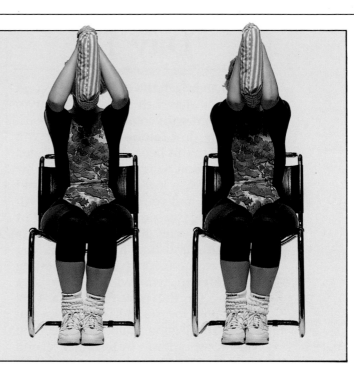

Vegetarian Menu Plan

BREAKFAST
4fl oz/120ml orange juice
1oz/30g slice toast spread with
2 teaspoons low-fat spread,
topped with
1 poached egg and
grilled tomatoes

LUNCH
1oz/30g pitta filled with
2 tablespoons peanut butter and
1 tomato
Dessert: 4oz/120g pineapple
7½ tablespoons low-fat natural yogurt

DINNER
4oz/120g smoked tofu, cooked in water with
1 vegetable stock cube, mixed with
cooked carrots, broccoli, onion, red and green pepper

8oz/240g potato
Dessert: Barbados Nutmeg Ice Cream (1 serving)

THROUGHOUT THE DAY
½ pint/300ml skimmed milk

BARBADOS NUTMEG ICE CREAM

¾ pint/450ml skimmed milk
1 vanilla pod or 1 teaspoon vanilla essence
1 teaspoon freshly ground nutmeg
3 eggs, beaten
6oz/180g plain fromage frais (8% fat)
artificial sweetener to taste

1 Heat the milk in a saucepan with the vanilla pod or essence and nutmeg until just below boiling point. Set aside to cool and infuse for 10 minutes.

2 Strain the flavoured milk on to the beaten eggs, whisk well and strain back into the saucepan. Heat very gently, stirring continuously until the sauce thickens.
3 Beat the fromage frais until smooth. Gradually mix in the custard sauce. Add sweetener to taste and pour into a rigid freezer container and freeze until almost firm.
4 Turn out into a chilled bowl and whisk to break down the ice crystals. Return to the container and freeze until firm. Place in the refrigerator for 15 minutes to soften slightly before serving.

Preparation: 20 minutes plus freezing time

Serves 6 *100 calories per serving*

Selections per serving: ¼ Milk, 1 Protein

Day 13

As you approach the end of your second week, you may well be feeling ready to experiment with some of the delicious, slimming, low-calorie recipes that you will find in this book. We have included a few for you to try this week to show you how easy low-calorie cooking can be for you and your family. It is a myth that dieting is boring. With a little effort from you, your dieting can be really interesting and fun! By this stage you will be eating foods that are interesting and different, you will be exercising perhaps for the first time in a long while, and you should really be beginning to feel good about yourself. You will almost certainly be feeling fitter and more confident and you should be proud of your efforts so far. No cream cake or chocolate bar is worth throwing all of your achievements so far out of the window!

BREAKFAST
4fl oz/120ml tomato juice
1oz/30g cereal (not sugar-coated)
¼ pint/150ml skimmed milk

LUNCH
2½ oz/75g sardines, warmed on
2 x 1oz/30g slices toast, spread with
1 teaspoon low-fat spread each
Dessert: 1 medium apple
2½fl oz/75ml low-fat natural yogurt

DINNER
beefburger with bun, filled with onion
2 teaspoons tomato ketchup
mixed salad
4 teaspoons low-calorie mayonnaise
Dessert: 3oz/90g grapes
1oz/30g hard cheese, e.g. Cheddar

THROUGHOUT THE DAY
½ pint/300ml skimmed milk

FOOD FOR THOUGHT
Many dieters find that it is the snacks between meals that they miss the most when they are watching their calorie intake. You will notice that we haven't itemized snacks specifically which can be eaten throughout the day, but you may of course save some of the meal ingredients to enjoy as a snack at any time. If you look at the foods we have suggested today, for example, you could have the yogurt from breakfast mixed with the chopped apple from lunch as a 4pm snack. As cereal can be eaten at any time, you may prefer to enjoy a bowl of cornflakes as an evening snack with milk from your daily allowance.

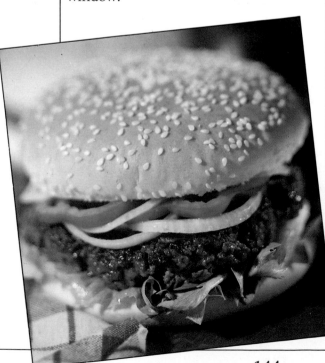

Aerobics

Now that you are getting fitter, how about introducing some aerobics? You will need a chair for this exercise. Stand a little distance away from it, and lean forwards with your hands resting on the seat of the chair. Keeping your stomach pulled in tightly, jump from leg

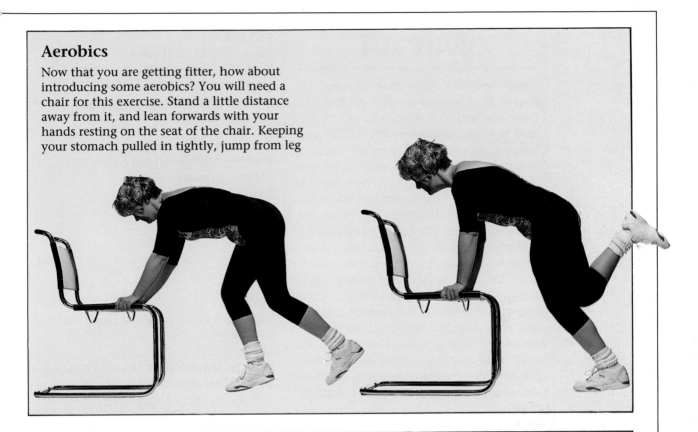

Vegetarian Menu Plan

BREAKFAST
6oz/180g strawberries
5fl oz/150ml low-fat natural yogurt
1oz/30g slice bread
2 teaspoons low-fat spread
1 boiled egg

LUNCH
1oz/30g pitta bread, spread with
1 tablespoon peanut butter
tomato, radish, mustard
and cress
Dessert: 2oz/60g pineapple

DINNER
6oz/180g cooked
pasta, mixed with
mushroom and onion, cooked in
1 teaspoon oil
6oz/180g soft tofu, cooked in stock with
carrots and cauliflower
4oz/120g peas
Dessert: Apricot and Orange Snow

THROUGHOUT THE DAY
½ pint/300ml skimmed milk

APRICOT AND ORANGE SNOW

6oz/180g drained canned apricots
½ tablespoon frozen concentrated orange juice, thawed
pinch of ground ginger or cinnamon
½ teaspoon caster sugar
1 egg white
pinch of cream of tartar

1 Mash the apricots with a fork.
2 Blend in the orange juice, ground spice and sugar.
3 Not more than 20 minutes before serving, whisk the egg white with the cream of tartar. Fold into the fruit purée and spoon into a dish.

Preparation: 10 minutes

Serves 1: *120 calories*

Selections: 1½ Fruit, 45 Optional Calories

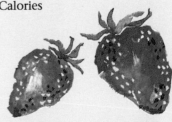

Day 14

Congratulations! You have reached the end of your second week! Now that you have reached this stage you can be sure that nothing will get in the way of your success. As you weigh yourself today to measure your weight loss, do try and think how different you feel now in comparison to two weeks ago when you embarked upon this personal challenge. Can you imagine just how good you will feel when you are even further towards your weight loss goal? You will now be able to plan your daily eating more closely around the foods that you enjoy but you can of course continue to use our meal suggestions as a framework if you wish. *Keep up the good work.* You can and will succeed. You are in total control and just remember . . . *take one day at a time . . . tomorrow will look after itself.*

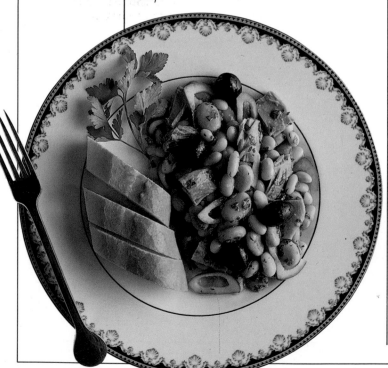

BREAKFAST
6fl oz/180ml fruit juice
½ oz/15g lean grilled back bacon
1 egg, scrambled in
2 teaspoons low-fat spread

LUNCH
2oz/60g tuna, mixed with
3oz/90g mixed canned beans
chopped onion
5 small olives, tossed in
1½ teaspoons oil
1 teaspoon vinegar
1oz/30g French bread
Dessert: 5fl oz/150ml low-fat natural yogurt

DINNER
3oz/90g cooked pork OR lamb OR beef
8oz/240g potato
cabbage, carrots, broccoli
Banana Honey Ice Cream (1 serving)
3fl oz/90ml sherry OR ½ pint/300ml beer, bitter, pale ale or cider

THROUGHOUT THE DAY
½ pint/300ml skimmed milk

FOOD FOR THOUGHT
If you like the occasional tipple, you will notice that at the end of each week we have included a small glass of sherry or wine or a ½ pint of beer or cider. These are completely optional. Alcohol has no nutritional qualities but lots of calories and in a way is rather like consuming liquid cream cakes!

Enjoyed now and again, the odd glass of wine will not ruin your diet but if the temptation is too much, omit it altogether until you are further down the path to successful slimming.

BANANA HONEY ICE CREAM

In our opinion, ice cream should always be made in bulk to make the most efficient use of the lengthy preparation time. However, a whole tub of ice cream in the freezer can be a dieter's nightmare. The beauty of this recipe is that it is intended for only two people or one dieter to enjoy twice.

1 tablespoon custard powder
⅓ pint/200ml skimmed milk
few drops of vanilla essence
½ medium banana
½ tablespoon clear honey
few drops of lemon juice
2 tablespoons whipping cream

1   Blend the custard powder with 1-2 tablespoons of milk. Bring the remaining milk and vanilla essence to the boil and stir into the blended custard powder. Return to the saucepan and heat gently to thicken, and then cook for 1 more minute.
2   Mash the banana, honey and lemon juice. Mix in the custard and transfer to a rigid container. Cool and then freeze until almost solid.
3   Turn out into a chilled bowl and whisk to break up the crystals. Whip the cream and whisk into the mixture. Return to the freezer in 2 individual containers until solid.
4   Place in the refrigerator for 10 minutes to soften before serving.

Preparation: 5 minutes plus freezing time
Cooking: 3 minutes
Serves 2 *140 calories per serving*
Selections per serving: ½ Fruit, 105 Optional Calories

Spinal stretch rotations

You could make this part of the cool-down sequence at the end of your home work-out. Lie on the floor with legs together and knees bent back to the right. Stretch your right arm out and back and bring your left arm across your body. Turn your head to the right and feel the stretch throughout your body. Hold for 20-30 seconds, breathing slowly, then swing over and repeat on other side.

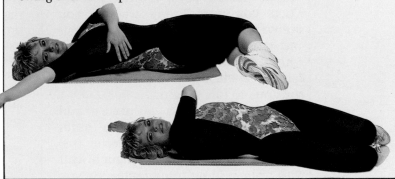

Upper body and buttocks stretch

Kneel down on all-fours and lower your head and outstretched arms all the way down to the floor. Stretch your body as far as feels comfortable, pulling back towards your feet, and hold for 20-30 seconds.

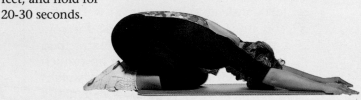

Vegetarian Menu Plan

BREAKFAST
4fl oz/120ml grapefruit juice
1oz/30g cereal
¼ pint/150ml skimmed milk

LUNCH
1oz/30g slice toast
6oz/180g baked beans
onion, watercress
2½fl oz/75ml low-fat natural yogurt

DINNER
1oz/30g vegetarian burger, cooked in
1½ teaspoons oil, topped with
1oz/30g slice cheese
8oz/240g potato
3oz/90g sweetcorn kernels
courgettes
Dessert: 1 medium orange
4fl oz/120ml wine

THROUGHOUT THE DAY
½ pint/300ml skimmed milk

At Weight Watchers, we like to think of weight maintenance as your third skill. You know what to eat to put on weight, and you have learned what to eat to lose weight. Now you will be able to acquire the vital third skill – how to maintain your target weight and stay slim.

Your starting point is what you ate when you were losing weight. You should have been eating sensible meals and snacks and you should continue with this, but you need to add some calories gradually so that you do not continue to lose weight.

In order to do this, you need to add some additional Selections (see pages 30-39) or extra Optional Calories (see page 40). You could try eating a biscuit with your mid-morning coffee, or you could treat yourself to an extra slice of toast or some fruit with your breakfast. Some people are so used to eating the food they enjoyed when they were losing weight that they continue eating the same things during the week, but relax and eat a little more at weekends. You must do whatever works for you.

By gradually introducing extra food in this way, you will discover how much you can eat without gaining any weight or losing further weight. It is all a matter of balance. If you sink below your target weight, you just need to add an additional Selection or two to add a few extra calories to your daily diet. If you go above it, you can cut back on these extra calories. Look at the graph on page 150 to help you; it is the easy way to monitor your weight and stay slim.

Mark your weight on the graph, or, if you don't like writing in this book, make a copy of the graph. Record your weight every week. In this way, you will soon discover exactly what you must eat

ANGELA WHITFIELD

Looking at Angela Whitfield now, it is hard to believe that she used to weigh nearly 16 stone. Angela reached her Goal Weight over three years ago. She had been overweight since her early childhood, but it was only after her marriage that the weight really began to pile on. Children followed, and she tried to lose weight in between the births of her two sons, Jonathan and Sam, but with little success. "I'd diet all week, really starve myself and lose a few pounds, but at the weekend I would binge and put it all on again."

Eventually, when she was 24, Angela was forced to admit that she had a dress size to match. "The most awful thing about being so fat was that I could only buy clothes from outsize shops. I used to look at other women going into chain stores and wonder how they could be that slim?"

Angela used to hide behind a facade of being happy and contented. "I used to laugh when friends tried to persuade me to diet, pretending that I didn't worry about my weight at all."

However, when a new friend commented on how 'jolly' Angela always was, she had a terrible vision of herself as a 'happy fat lady from a freak show or circus'. She knew that she had to do something about her weight, and when

to maintain your weight. Don't worry if your weight fluctuates within one or two pounds on either side of your target weight – this is normal.

Successful weight maintenance

The secret is balance: eating a healthy balanced diet, and balancing the energy

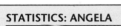

STATISTICS: ANGELA
AGE: 29
HEIGHT: 5 feet 6 inches
WAS: 15 stone 11 pounds
NOW: 9 stone
LOST: 6 stone 11 pounds

she passed her driving test, the first place she drove to was her local Weight Watchers Meeting.

Angela has never looked back since. It took just seven months for her to shed nearly 7 stone, and trade in her shapeless dresses for a new size 10 wardrobe. She really enjoys the Programme, and even now she still goes to Meetings once a month working as a clerk for the Leader. "It helps to keep me on the straight and narrow, and I still pick up useful tips."

Angela has found it relatively easy to stay at her Goal Weight, just by adopting a more healthy low-fat diet. Losing weight has changed her whole life. "I'm much more confident and willing to give anything a go. The only thing I regret is that I wasted so much time being unhappy and overweight."

She got a job as a beauty assistant for a top cosmetics company, something she would never have dreamed of applying for when she was overweight. Life has become more fun, and her favourite saying is "Nothing tastes as good as being slim feels!"

your body gets in the form of food with the amount of energy it burns. You can compare it with a healthy bank account. If you spend more than you earn, you will go into debit and will have problems. However, if you spend less than you earn, you will be in credit. In the same way, if you eat a little less in the week and keep some in reserve, you can treat yourself at weekends.

Exercise will also help you to stay at your target weight (see page 155) and brings many benefits. The more you exercise, the more food you will be able to eat and still maintain your weight.

One thing that you should have learned from our Programme is a healthier, better way to eat. You now know which are the best foods for your weight and your health, and which ones are

LBS	Your Staying Slim Graph						Action Needed
GW + 7							Cut out 20 additional Selections and 500 Optional Calories this week
GW + 6							Cut out 16 additional Selections and 400 Optional Calories this week
GW + 5							Cut out 12 additional Selections and 300 Optional Calories this week
GW + 4							Cut out 8 additional Selections and 200 Optional Calories this week
GW + 3							Cut out 4 additional Selections and 100 Optional Calories this week
GW + 2							**Your weight is fine.** Eat the same number of Selections, additional Selections and Optional Calories as last week Continue with the same level of exercise activity
GW + 1							
Goal Weight							
GW – 1							
GW – 2							Add 4 additional Selections and 100 Optional Calories this week
GW – 3							Add 8 additional Selections and 200 Optional Calories this week
GW – 4							Add 12 additional Selections and 300 Optional Calories this week
GW – 5							Add 16 additional Selections and 400 Optional Calories this week
GW – 6							Add 20 additional Selections and 500 Optional Calories this week
GW – 7							
	Week 1	Week 2	Week 3	Week 4	Week 5	Week 6	

To find out what you should eat to stay in control of your weight mark your weight on the graph. If you gain weight, cut out the additional Selections and Optional Calories stated (see page 148). If you lose weight, add additional Selections and Optional Calories as shown. The more you exercise, the more food you can eat – within reason.

best avoided. What you must not do is go back to your old eating habits and eat too many of those foods that made you overweight in the first place. Of course, you can't continue eating exactly the same as when you were losing weight or your weight may fall below the acceptable level at the bottom of the healthy weight range (see page 13) specified for your age, height and sex.

So what should you do?
Knowing the problems that many of our successful Members face, we have created a special Maintenance Programme to help you stay slim. You still eat the wide range of foods that you enjoyed on our weight loss Programme, but you can relax the rules a little.

Some of our Members find that it is a great relief not to have to follow a food plan, and they enjoy the ability to choose larger portions of foods, or snacks, more often. However, others find it very difficult to adapt and to make sensible food choices when shopping and planning their meals. It is so tempting to reach out for items on supermarket shelves that they have denied themselves for so long.

Our advice to you is that the odd treat will do no harm and that no foods are forbidden – again, it is all a matter of getting the balance right. If you go out to a restaurant or a friend's house for dinner and treat yourself to a creamy dessert or an extra glass of wine, don't worry, because you can just cut down on something the following day to

ANNE SEWELL

Anne Sewell has not only lost over 3 stone but she has also successfully stayed slim. It is two years since Anne reached her Goal Weight and achieved her size 12 shape. Now she is a Weight Watchers Leader, helping other members to achieve their ambitions.

Before Anne went to Weight Watchers, she had been battling with her weight for years, since she became pregnant with her first child. "I was one of those lucky people who could eat more or less whatever I wanted without gaining a pound; that is, until after the birth of my daughter, Joanne. It was such a shock when I was left with an extra stone that I found impossible to shift. By the time I had my second daughter, Janet, seventeen months later, I was 2 stone overweight."

Anne's sedentary job as a liaison officer with a fashion company didn't help, and she gained another stone. By the time she joined Weight Watchers, she was 3 stone overweight, but it took only five months for her to shed this and reach her goal. Being slim and becoming a Leader has made an enormous difference to her lifestyle. "There just isn't enough time in the day to overeat. I eat the same food as everyone else because Weight Watchers food is normal food. I don't over-indulge and I make sure I never feel deprived."

Anne thinks that the trick of staying slim, especially when it comes to special occasions, is to plan for your favourite treat so you can enjoy it without feeling an ounce of guilt. "For example, at Christmas, a lot of my Members enjoy a few tipples, so I suggest having one alcoholic drink at the beginning of the evening, then drinking sparkling water so that they can look forward to another

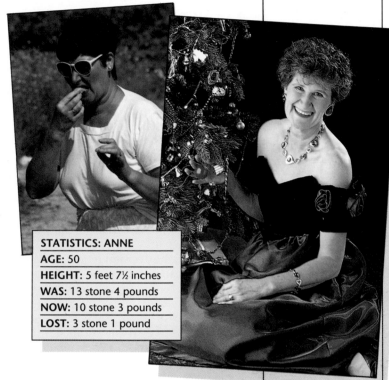

STATISTICS: ANNE
AGE: 50
HEIGHT: 5 feet 7½ inches
WAS: 13 stone 4 pounds
NOW: 10 stone 3 pounds
LOST: 3 stone 1 pound

glass of wine, or whatever, later on. It's easy if you plan what you're going to eat and drink."

Anne points out that you don't have to be a fitness fanatic to keep in shape; there are other ways of keeping fit and building some exercise into your everyday lifestyle. "I used to think exercise was a dirty word until I realised that gardening was toning me up as much as any aerobics class. Even if you just use the stairs instead of the lift, and get up to switch TV channels instead of using the remote control, you'll burn up some extra calories."

Anne's shining example proves that you can stay slim successfully just by eating sensibly, staying active and exercising in moderation. It's not difficult to find the right balance that works for you.

MARK PEAK

When Mark was 11 years old, he was taller and fatter than the other children, which was hard when all he wanted was to mingle with everyone else and be accepted as 'normal'. His weight made him depressed, and he made the mistake of turning to food for comfort, so much so that by the time he was 19 he weighed over 19 stone. Mark was then faced with the impossible task of trying to buy trendy clothes that would fit, and compensated for being the butt of jokes by being the life and soul of the party instead.

For Mark, the decision to join Weight Watchers came when he and four friends, all overweight, sat down to huge plates of pies, chips and curry, plus a few lagers. One of them said that they looked as if they'd all escaped from Weight Watchers! "We suddenly realised we were absolutely huge. Then someone suggested we really should join Weight Watchers before we all died of

heart attacks – and we made a pact."

A year later, Mark had lost over five stone and had won the title of Photogenic Ambassador in the Weight Watchers Success of the Year 1991 competition. He says: "I've now got a better job as a Senior Social Worker. I looked good and felt good when I went for the interview, and I think that's what came across. Different types of people talk to me now. Before I lost weight, some people would never have given me the time of day."

Mark is now completely in control of his eating habits. Long gone are the days when he used to get pleasure from feeling full and bloated. "Now if I eat too much it feels awful – but that's how it used to be all the time. It's nice now to feel light." He still allows himself the occasional treat, especially Indian food, but this is his only indulgence as he has given up drinking lager and is now completely teetotal. "I'm saving all that money and I'm still going out and having a really good time."

Mark now feels more confident in himself and in his clothes. He now walks tall instead of slouching in the hope of making himself less noticeable. In fact, his whole life has changed since he made the decision to join Weight Watchers.

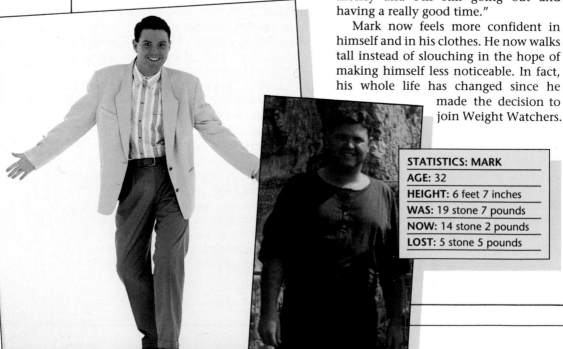

STATISTICS: MARK	
AGE: 32	
HEIGHT: 6 feet 7 inches	
WAS: 19 stone 7 pounds	
NOW: 14 stone 2 pounds	
LOST: 5 stone 5 pounds	

compensate. No harm has been done. If you make a habit of overeating and do it regularly, then you are bound to put on some weight.

You can still eat lots of food and you will never go hungry. By now, vegetables, skimmed milk and low-fat products should be the norm and an important part of your daily food. In fact, if you spread some butter too thickly on your toast, or sugar your coffee overgenerously, or have a huge helping of whipped cream on your fruit salad, you may not even enjoy the taste any more. Many of our Members who have lost weight successfully on the Programme say that their food preferences have changed. For example, some have begun to enjoy the true flavour and aroma of black coffee and tea; by adding sugar, all they can taste is the sugar which overpowers the real flavour. When your tastebuds have become accustomed to a less sweet, less fatty diet, then you will feel like this too and won't crave foods that are high in fat and sugar as often.

Balancing the calories

We have already discovered that we lose weight when we take in fewer calories than we burn. So in order to maintain our weight we have to balance the number of calories we eat and the number we burn. In this way, we will neither lose nor gain weight. This is not as difficult to achieve as you might think. You do not have to count calories religiously – that is not the Weight Watchers way and is only likely to make you obsessive about your weight and what you eat. Our attitude is more relaxed. All you need do is to follow the guidelines laid down in our Programme, which should be automatic by now.

Maintenance guidelines

- Make sure you eat a variety of foods from the different food groups
- Continue eating plenty of vegetables from the list on page 119 to fill you up and stop you feeling hungry
- If you feel like a snack, eat vegetables, fruit, crispbreads and low-fat products
- Avoid fatty foods and fry-ups
- Limit the amount of sugar in your tea, coffee and other hot drinks
- Keep chocolate, biscuits and sweets as treats rather than everyday foods
- Choose fresh fruit or low-fat yogurt for desserts
- Always use skimmed milk in preference to full-fat milk
- Continue eating chicken and white fish in preference to red meat
- If you do eat red meat or bacon, carefully remove all fat
- Opt for reduced-calorie dressings, mayonnaise and other food products
- Choose low-fat spreads in preference to butter
- Use low-fat natural or fruit yogurt instead of cream as a topping for desserts
- Use artificial sweetener as a sweetening agent, if desired

Remember
- You are not dieting any more; try to achieve a balance
- Eat a *little* more food than when you were losing weight
- Try to exercise regularly
- Energy output must balance food intake

- Beware of hidden calories, i.e. fats and sugars, in processed foods; always read the labels carefully
- Make sure you eat plenty of high-fibre foods, such as whole-grain cereals, fruit, beans and vegetables. Foods high in fibre are filling and satisfying
- Use skimmed milk when making rice puddings, pancakes, Yorkshire puddings, white sauces and hot drinks
- Don't overeat. Your motto should be 'everything in moderation'. That slice of quiche or cake might taste delicious but you don't have to eat the whole thing
- Don't eat alone or in secret. Always eat with other members of your family if possible in a relaxed atmosphere and stick to your pattern of three meals a day: breakfast, light meal and main meal. Then you are less likely to feel hungry and be tempted to snack on foods you haven't planned for
- Don't be afraid of refusing food for fear of offending someone. If you explain, they *will* understand
- Learn to be 'menu-literate' when you eat out so that you can recognise the healthier, less fattening choices
- Do not drink too much wine, beer or spirits. Not only are they high in calories, but they may also diminish your will power
- Continue drinking plenty of water every day. It contains no calories, it helps fill you up and flushes out and cleanses your body
- If you must drink fizzy drinks, opt for low-calorie versions
- Don't drink too much fruit juice; it should never be drunk freely like water, as fruit contains natural sugars and can add unwanted calories to your diet
- Don't eat too many eggs; the yolks are high in cholesterol. You should not eat more than seven eggs per week
- Don't shop when you are hungry
- Keep a look-out for new low-fat and low-sugar products to try
- Lastly, don't worry! All of these guidelines will soon become second nature to you. In the end, sensible eating boils down to common sense and putting into practice what you have learned on our Programme

Lifestyle changes

You may think that the only things that affect your weight are how much you eat and how much you exercise, but there are other factors too. You may have been doing a good job of maintaining your weight, but suddenly you start putting it on again. Often this is due to a lifestyle change: maybe you have changed your job and are doing more sedentary work – sitting behind a desk all day and getting less exercise.

Of course, a lifestyle change can cause you to lose weight too. If you enjoy exercising and feeling fitter, and step up your level and frequency of exercise, you may lose weight even if you are eating the same amount of food.

Fashion fax
- When you reach your target weight, take a photo of yourself to inspire you. You might even consider going to a professional photographer for an extra-special result. If you find that you are gaining weight again, you will be able to take a look at that photograph for the encouragement you need
- Treat yourself to a new dress or a pair of jeans and stay that shape

PAMELA VAILL

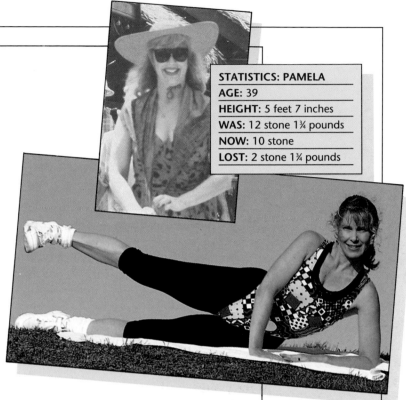

STATISTICS: PAMELA	
AGE: 39	
HEIGHT: 5 feet 7 inches	
WAS: 12 stone 1¾ pounds	
NOW: 10 stone	
LOST: 2 stone 1¾ pounds	

Pam Vaill's life has changed completely since she arrived in London from America, two stone overweight, to take up a job in the home video industry. Unfortunately that job fell through, but now, fit and slim, she is a personal fitness trainer and aerobics teacher.

Pam became very depressed when her promised job didn't materialize. She was stranded in a strange country looking for work, and the weight started piling on. She decided to take stock of her life and joined her local dance studio. She also took the decision to join Weight Watchers. "I had belonged to Meetings in the States, and had always managed to achieve my Goal Weight before slipping back into my old ways. I was determined that I would reach my goal this time and stay in shape."

Pam enjoyed the meetings, cooked all the recommended meals, and the weight started to shift. An instructor at the dance studio asked her to stand in for her while she was away, and that led to a new career. When Pam reached her goal, she was so delighted with her transformation that she decided to become a Weight Watchers Leader and now runs several weekly Meetings.

Healthy eating and regular exercise have both contributed to Pam's success. Her work as an aerobics instructor keeps her in great shape.

Staying slim

You now know how much food you need to eat to lose weight, and you are discovering how much you need to maintain your target weight and stay slim. The simple formula is: eat too many calories and you gain weight; too few and you lose weight. However, staying slim is more than just what you eat – it is important that you exercise regularly too.

If you have been following the exercise programme in this book, then exercise is probably becoming part of your usual routine. You mustn't stop now just because you have lost weight; it is more important than ever that you improve your fitness to maintain your new slim shape.

Follow the safety guidelines set down on page 100, to protect your health. You need to exercise for 20 minutes at least three times a week to enjoy the benefits of improved fitness. If you have not exercised a great deal in the past, it is best to start off with a gentle low-intensity activity, such as walking, swimming, cycling or our special exercise programme, which will all help to maintain your weight and firm up any slack muscles or problem areas like hips and thighs.

Walking

This is probably the best and easiest exercise of all. You can do it anywhere, anytime; you don't need special equipment; and it doesn't cost anything. Walking helps to burn up calories, increase your stamina and improve the efficiency of your heart and lungs. It is great cardiovascular exercise, improving circulation and lowering blood pressure. In order to get the most out of walking, you need to do it briskly. Try to build a little walking into your daily routine, gradually going a little further as you feel fitter. Rest if you feel weary or breathless, but if you try to keep moving you will improve your general circulation. Far from feeling tired at the end of a walk, you should feel invigorated and more energetic. Try to create opportunities for walking:

● Leave the car behind when you pop out to the local shops, visit a friend or go to work

● Walk the dog more often

● Go for family walks in the countryside or your local park

● Go for a walk in your lunch break

● Try hiking over rough terrain rather than a smooth road; it can increase your energy output by almost one-third

● Walk downhill: this sounds odd but it requires more skill than walking on level ground and uses more energy

Swimming

The buoyancy of water reduces your body weight by 90 per cent when you are swimming, thereby making it virtually impact- and stress-free. Like walking, it is another good cardiovascular exercise and helps to improve muscle tone and streamline your figure. It also develops stamina and suppleness.

You can just swim a few lengths or you can try working out in the water; this is one of the safest exercises of all. Because the water makes you 'weightless', your muscles can work more freely and you put less strain on your body. Many leisure centres with swimming pools hold special pool exercise classes, or 'aquarobics'. If you enjoy working out with other people, they might be worth considering. They are good fun and you can exercise safely under the supervision of a qualified instructor.

Other forms of exercise

The most important thing is to choose a sport or exercise that you *enjoy*. Then you will stick with it and receive all the benefits it brings: a stronger heart, increased flexibility, greater stamina, and a general well-being.

If you start off gradually by walking, swimming or following our work-out programme, then as you get fitter you can progress to more strenuous activities.

Exercising regularly can add a whole new dimension to your life and introduce you to new stimulating pastimes and new friends. If you have spent the last few years feeling overweight and not daring to break out, it is very liberating to take up a sport. As you strengthen your heart, burn up calories, tone up your muscles and help increase your metabolic rate, you can really enjoy yourself and enhance your quality of life.

Healthy eating to last a lifetime

By sticking to your new-found healthy eating habits you will find staying slim now easier than ever. By now you should be grilling, steaming and poaching instead of roasting and frying your food. You should know the difference between a healthy, nutritious snack and a high-calorie one. You should be choosing low-fat foods instinctively. You know that you can eat, and enjoy, a really varied diet without reverting back to the bad old days and gaining weight.

If you continue weighing yourself once a week and checking waist, hip and thigh measurements you can measure your success and learn how much food and which ones you can eat without putting on any weight. You will soon become more confident and it will be second nature to you to maintain your weight.

Don't make the mistake of thinking that you can eat exactly the same as your partner, family or friends. They may be taller or more energetic than you, and anyway no two bodies are the same, and it is a fact of life that some people can eat more than others. You have to find the right balance for you.

Maintenance menus

Here are some typical maintenance menus for you to try. Eat the food and recipes listed here, and you will have a better idea of how much you need to eat to maintain your target weight. If you find that you are dipping below it, you

should add a snack or a few calories to your daily plan. If you are rising above it, you could try omitting something, such as an ice cream or jelly dessert, to reduce your intake by a few calories. This may be enough to strike the right balance.

Maintenance menus

BREAKFAST

½ medium banana	**OR** ½ medium grapefruit	**OR** 4fl oz/120ml
1oz/30g cereal	1oz/30g slice toast	orange juice
½ pint/300ml milk	1 boiled egg	crispbread up
from daily		to 80 calories
allowance		2oz/60g low-fat soft cheese

LUNCH

2oz/60g chunk	**OR** 1oz/30g slices toast	**OR** 1 standard
French bread	2 teaspoons low-fat	pitta
2 teaspoons low-fat spread	spread	2 teaspoons
1oz/30g cheese	3oz/90g baked beans	low-fat spread
tomato, onion,	mushrooms	1 hard-boiled
cucumber	1 kiwi fruit	egg
1 medium apple		mixed salad
		3oz/90g grapes

DINNER

Chilli Chicken	**OR** Mixed Fish	**OR** 2oz/60g
Stir-fry	Casserole	vegetarian
(see page 76)	(see page 73)	sausage
6oz/180g cooked	6oz/180g cooked	8oz/240g
rice	rice or pasta	potato
mixed salad	mixed salad	3oz/90g
2oz/60g vanilla	4 teaspoons salad	baked beans
or strawberry	dressing	onion, cauli-
ice cream	¼ pint/150ml	flower
	prepared fruit	4 teaspoons
	flavoured jelly	tomato
		ketchup
		5fl oz/150ml
		very low-fat
		fruit yogurt

Every day use either: 1 pint/600ml skimmed milk **OR**
½ pint/300ml skimmed milk *and* 5fl oz/ 150ml low-fat natural yogurt **OR**
10 fl oz/300ml low-fat natural yogurt

Useful information

If you require further help or details of local Weight Watchers classes, please call us on 0628 777077 or contact your nearest Regional Centre as listed below. Or you can contact Weight Watchers By Mail on 091 296 2200.

1 Aberdeen. Tel: 0224 626171.
2 Altrincham. Tel: 061 929 0667.
3 Bicester. Tel: 0869 320411.
4 Birmingham. Tel: 021 233 2383.
5 Bristol. Tel: 0454 619799.
6 Cambridge. Tel: 0223 863233.
7 Cardiff. Tel: 0222 220525.
8 Cheshunt. Tel: 0992 24125.
9 Coventry. Tel: 0203 257122.
10 Edinburgh. Tel: 031 229 7111.
11 Exeter. Tel: 0392 824141.
12 Glasgow. Tel: 041 429 7373.
13 Harlow. Tel: 0279 433288.
14 Horsham. Tel: 0403 271749.
15 Leeds. Tel: 0532 452423.
16 Central London. Tel: 071 491 1929.
17 Maidenhead. Tel: 0628 777235.
18 Maidstone. Tel: 0622 683573.
19 Manchester. Tel: 061 228 6537.
20 Newark. Tel: 0636 612113.
21 Newcastle-on-Tyne.
    Tel: 091 461 0123.
22 Newcastle-under-Lyme.
    Tel: 0782 711072.
23 Preston. Tel: 0772 201456.
24 Romford. Tel: 0708 743311.
25 Sheffield. Tel: 0742 751061.
26 Southampton. Tel: 0703 63995.
27 St. Helens. Tel: 0744 30622.
28 Stockton. Tel: 0642 615317.
29 York. Tel: 0904 610678.

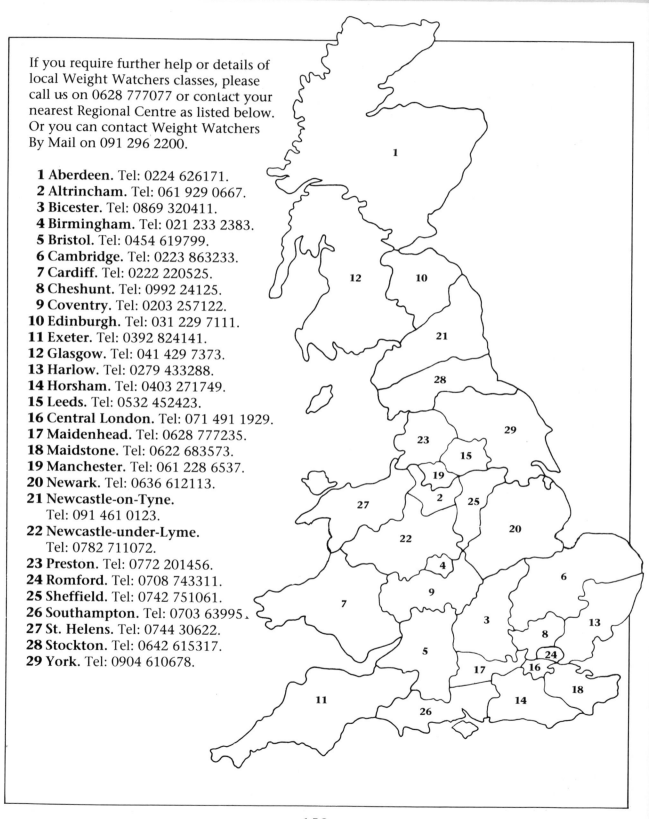

Index

RECIPE INDEX